AF884763

From Our Coaches' Kitchens

Ketolicious for Lipedema
Holiday Cookbook

Dedicated to each & everyone of YOU
our Lipedema Tribe.
You inspire us, we love you!

From Our Coaches' Kitchens

Ketolicious for Lipedema Holiday Cookbook

Lipedema Simplified Publications
The Lipedema Project
Lipedema-Simplified.org

AUTHORS

Megan Pfeffer, Mende Staggs, Catherine A. Seo,
Raeann Sparks, Brenda Gold, Carol Rowsemitt, Leslyn Keith

FROM OUR COACHES' KITCHENS: KETOLICIOUS FOR LIPEDEMA HOLIDAY COOKBOOK

PUBLISHED BY:
Lipedema Simplified Publications
The Lipedema Project
60 Boston Ave
Somerville, MA 02144 United States
+1-617-721-9463
https://Lipedema-Simplified.org/

Permission for Use

Citation

Pfeffer, M., Staggs, M., Seo, C. A., Sparks, R., Gold, B., Rowsemitt, C., & Keith, L. (2019). *From our coaches' kitchens: Ketolicious for lipedema holiday cookbook.* Boston, MA: Lipedema Simplified Publications.

As appropriate for digital use include the following:
© Lipedema Simplified. 2019. Used with permission.
for more information https://Lipedema-Simplified.org/

Layout & Design: Lipedema Simplified Publishing
Photos: Adobe Images, iStock, Raeann Sparks
Editors: Megan Pfeffer, BHSc and Catherine A. Seo, PhD

ISBN: 978-0-9989845-3-7 (print edition)

Library of Congress Control Number: *Application in process*
Publication date: November 2019
Printed in the United States of America.

Keto Caveat

Note: This book is a relaxed and realistic approach to keto throughout the holidays for special celebrations. This gives you the option of tailoring the recipes to your individual responses to food and provides the option to include foods that can be celebratory, with an emphasis on the recipes being for special occasions.

These recipes are better/healthier alternatives to non-keto foods and are not recommended as everyday food choices. We find that including these options supports consistently staying in nutritional ketosis throughout challenging social events while encouraging a balanced and self-caring approach to our food. When choosing to eat these special occasion foods, total daily carbs should stay below 50 g per day with optimal carbs below 20 g (total) per day.

Ketolicious Table of Contents

Merry
delicious
and
blessed

Ketolicious Holidays!

"Love is not only the most important ingredient:
it is the only ingredient that really matters."

~Edward Espe Brown (from a cookbook by a British chef)

Welcome to Ketolicious for the Holidays!

My favorite book of all time is "*The Tassajara Bread Book*" by Edward Espe Brown. Tassajara Zen Mountain Center is nestled deep in a valley by hot springs in the Ventana Wilderness, within the Santa Lucia Range and Los Padres National Forest in Monterey County, California. Edward Espe Brown was the kitchen master and chef when I visited there in the early 1970s.

I've had my original copy from 1971 for almost 50 years, even though I've traveled and lived in many places, packed, unpacked, repacked many times, and most especially that I haven't eaten bread since 1987 when starting my low carbohydrate (low carb) journey. The cover is coming off, many pages are discolored and stained from baking ingredients from so many years ago. Still, when I pick it up and go through its pages, I am reminded of the most fundamental truth. *Food is nurturing and meant to add to our lives, to give pleasure and sustenance. The love, respect, honor, and deeply sacred relationship possible with food is an intimate connection meant to offer life, nourishment, and health.*

I am one who has strayed far and wide and ardently struggled with listening to my body and discovering the right food plan for me. I am a bit in awe to share that a ketogenic way of eating has been the light at the end of a very long and arduous journey.

The Promise of Ketolicious

This cookbook and the recipes here are offered to allow you to enjoy the holidays while staying in ketosis. Ketosis is the precious gift of a ketogenic lifestyle, the ability of our bodies to switch into fat-burning from sugar/glucose burning. Ketosis is explained further by our clinical nutritionist, Megan Pfeffer, below.

The reason we wrote this cookbook is to offer options so that you can choose to stay in ketosis while enjoying holiday fare. You CAN eat luxuriously while taking care of yourself, your health, your body, and your lipedema/lymphatic disorder. Keto offers promise for so many of us in managing lipedema, lymphedema, and lymphatic & fat disorders. We find that inflammation disappears, swelling diminishes, the pain goes away - and the miracle of miracles - many of us lose weight. All while eating delicious and luxurious food. This can accompany us throughout the holidays. These festive occasions can also be a time of enjoyment and self-care.

Our coaches have all personally transformed their lives with a ketogenic lifestyle along with other conservative measures. Several have lost and maintained 70-100+ pounds while creating foods that satisfy and are KETOLICIOUS! We coach and consult with lipedema ladies and healthcare providers worldwide to support the same transformative lifestyles for others as well. We serve as faculty facilitating our MasterClasses (6-month intensive support groups) and our Mini-MasterClasses (2-month quick-start support groups).

While at one time it was commonly thought that lipedema fat is "resistant to diet and exercise" the early research of Leslyn Keith, OTD, CLT-LANA, opened the door to prove otherwise. Thousands of those with lymphatic/fat disorders are now reporting life-enhancing results. Truly, keto for lipedema/lymphatic disorders is a game-changer.

We recommend simple food and simply delicious eating as a lifestyle. Several of these recipes are for festive occasions and not for day-to-day fare. Our goal is to offer choices to support you in maintaining your ketosis so you can stay healthy and happy throughout the holidays! We hope this expands your options. Nothing is impossible!

Ketolicious on!

With much love!

Catherine

Catherine A. Seo, PhD
Director & Founder
Lipedema Simplified
The Lipedema Project
Lipedema-Simplified.org
catherine@lipedema-simplified.org

About Our Coaching Program

Lipedema is a complex fat and lymphatic disorder that affects every aspect of our lives: physical, mental/psychological, emotional, spiritual, and social. Lipedema and weight can show up very differently in each of us. One nutrition plan doesn't work for everyone. We have found that a customized and personalized plan to manage your lipedema works for many lipedema ladies.

Online Support Group

Keto Way of Eating for Lipedema on Facebook

We started a Facebook support group in 2016. It's going strong today with close to 8,900 members. We actively support a keto lifestyle and encourage bio-hacking keto so it fits your situation like a glove. You are welcome to join us! https://www.facebook.com/groups/LipedemaKetoWOE/

Why Coaching & Mentoring?

Because we are each unique.

No two women have the same situation, stage, type, various comorbidities, and other things that impact our health. Lipedema can't be treated by a formula, instead we have found that a customized and personalized plan to manage lipedema and lose weight works for many lipedema ladies. That's why working with the right coach is invaluable.

We support bio-individuality by partnering with you to discover what's right for you. Our team approach allows us to consult with one another to help you craft the program that's right for you. You can work with one coach knowing that you have the entire team consulting as needed.

Any of our coaches are happy to chat with you to see if we can help and if it might be the right next step for you. For more information about our coaches and coaching program: https://lipedema-simplified.org/coaching/

Our Authors & Coaching Team

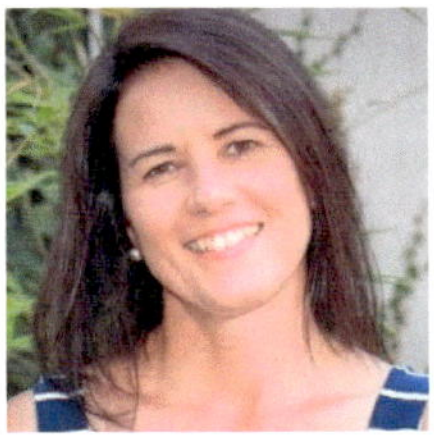

Megan Pfeffer, BHSc is a degree qualified Clinical Nutritionist, with a Bachelor of Health Science in Nutritional & Dietetic Medicine. Megan specializes in LCHF (low carbohydrate high fat) and ketogenic lifestyles for the management of health and chronic disease. Megan follows a ketogenic lifestyle herself to manage her own Lipedema.

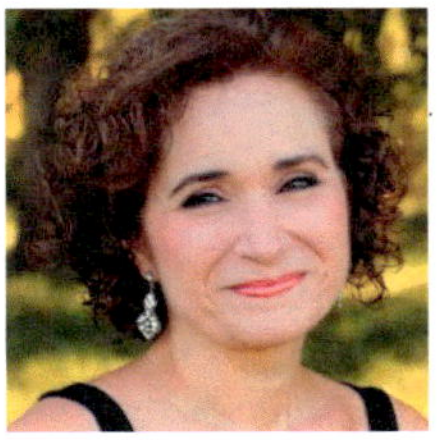

Mende Staggs is a keto chef and coach. She specializes in cooking & culinary arts. After finding great success in managing her lipedema and migraine headaches with the ketogenic way of eating, Mende is using her cooking and teaching experience to coach women with lipedema in the keto lifestyle. Mende has completed the Professional Training in LCHF/Ketogenic Nutrition and Treatment with The Noakes Foundation.

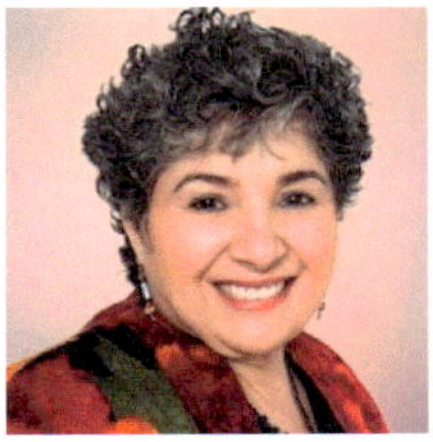

Catherine Seo, PhD is Director, lipedema Simplified and The lipedema Project. She produced and directed the documentary, *The Disease They Call FAT,* and was a co-author of the book, *Lipedema-The Disease They Call FAT: An Overview for Clinicians*. Her research focuses on empowering women applying self-compassion meditation techniques. Dr. Seo follows a keto way of eating, intermittent fasting and carnivore to manage her own lipedema and lymphedema.

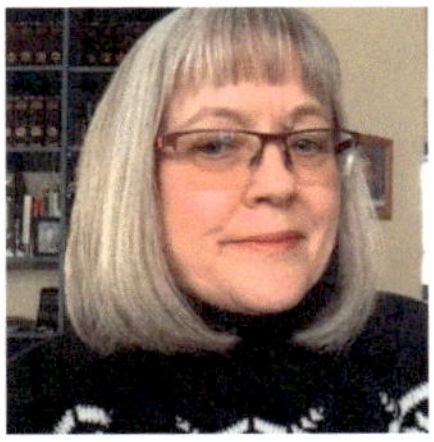

Raeann Sparks, BFA, BEd is a Teacher and Certified Keto Coach. Lipedema put her in a wheelchair. She used Keto, Intermittent Fasting (IF), Extended Fasting (EF), cortisone injections, pool exercise, swimming, compression, and cycling to walk unaided again. Her Ketogenic Way of Eating also remitted her type 2 Diabetes. Raeann has completed the Professional Training in LCHF/Ketogenic Nutrition and Treatment with The Noakes Foundation.

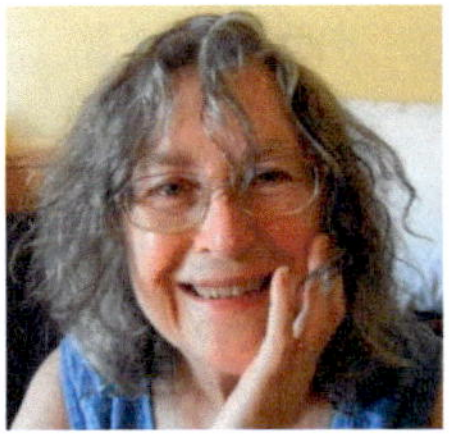

Brenda Gold, BHSc, (PT) is a physiotherapist and coach. Brenda joined our MasterClass dealing with the loss of her husband plus several other co-morbidities in addition to lipedema. She found "releasing" especially helpful so continued to the teacher training. She has been coaching & helping others in "letting go" of emotional blocks and flowing into greater freedom.

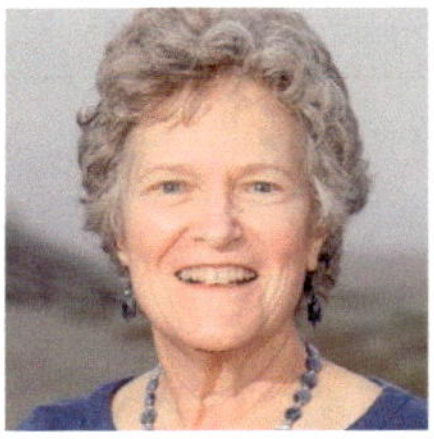

Carol "Rosey" Rowsemitt, PhD, RN, FNP is a family nurse practitioner. She specializes in weight management and understands that the famine response often increases appetite and decreases metabolism to protect against weight loss when food is insufficient. She assesses and treats famine response hypothyroidism. This dual-pronged approach helps patients lose weight and keep it off.

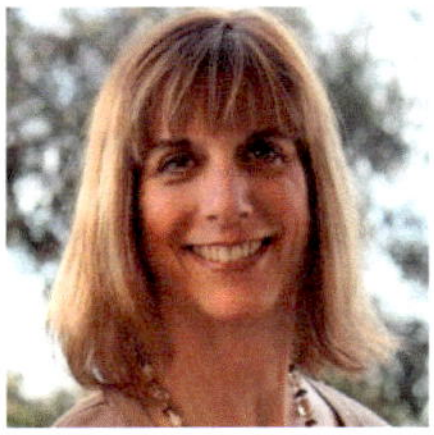

Leslyn Keith, OTD, CLT-LANA is Director of Research for The Lipedema Project, an instructor in lymphedema therapy for Klose Training and Consulting and has a private practice in lymphedema/lipedema therapy. She is the author of the recently released book, *The Ketogenic Solution for Lymphatic Disorders.* Dr. Keith's research is groundbreaking, and she is considered an expert in nutrition for lymphatic disorders. She presents at conferences worldwide.

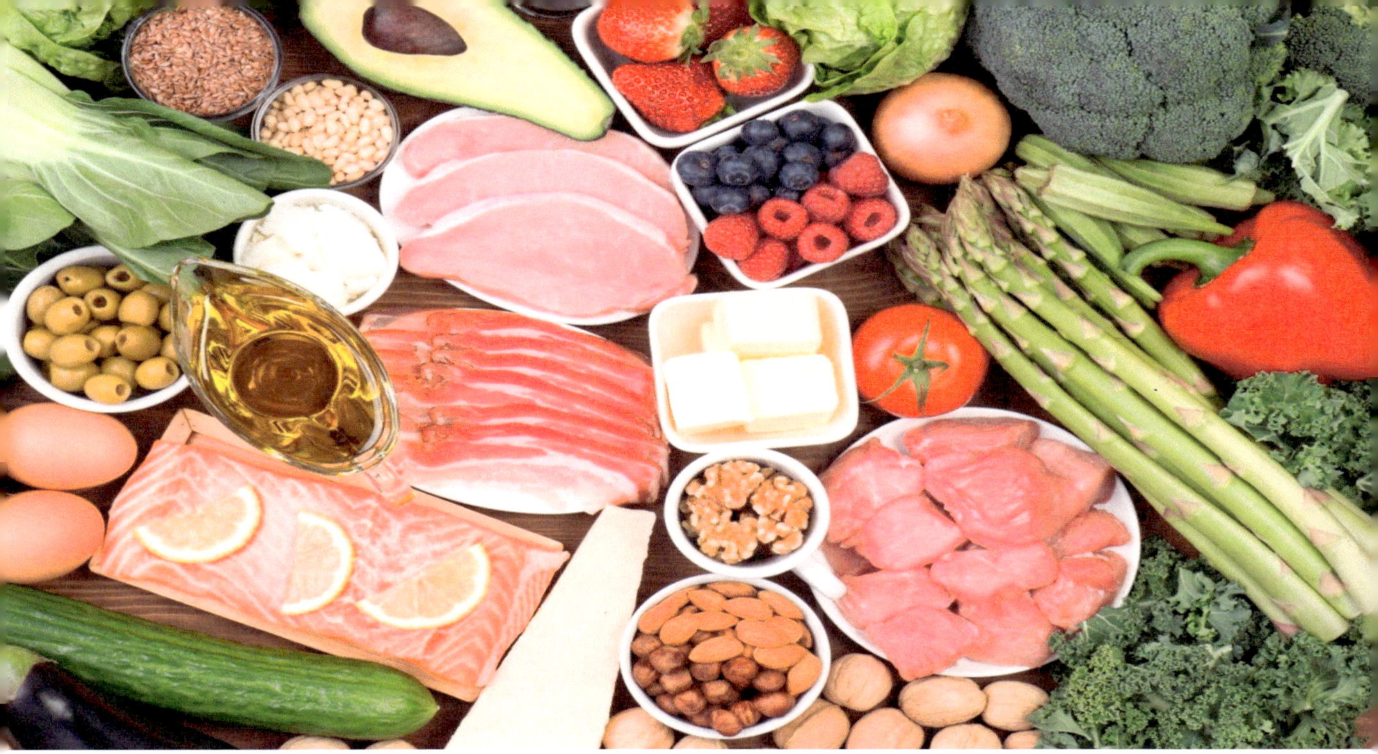

From Our Nutritionist

The keto recipes in this book are delicious, decadent and perfect for the holiday season. They contain plenty of wholesome, nutrient dense foods as well as desserts for special occasions. You can happily enjoy the food festivities and meet your keto macro targets, all while consuming a good variety of nutritious foods.

Of course, the holidays are also for spending quality time with family and friends and building community spirit, so ultimately if you are staying in nutritional ketosis during this busy time, then well done! Concentrating further on nutrient dense foods and food intolerances are too much for some over the holidays but a great health bonus for others - we are all different in our approach to the festive season and it is, after all, important to relax and reduce stress to improve health and enjoy the holidays.

One of the most important things to keep in mind when it comes to food and our health is that we are all different and unique. No two people will react to food in exactly the same way, and we need to consider this when working out our approach to diet and lifestyle.

I follow a ketogenic (keto) diet to manage my lipedema, and I continue this throughout the holidays. There are so many amazing recipes nowadays to make staying in ketosis easily achievable, and I always feel quite proud of myself for prioritizing my health and creating new festive food favorites. Out with the old, in with the new!

About Nutritional Ketosis

Nutritional ketosis is defined as having a blood ketone reading of 0.5 mmol/L or above. Ensuring you are well versed in the art and science of following a well-formulated ketogenic diet, in addition to speaking with your doctor about the impact of dietary changes on your medical condition/s and medication/s, prior to eating keto foods will help to avoid common pitfalls such as electrolyte imbalance, low blood sugar and low blood pressure. Eating high fat keto food if you are still on a high carbohydrate diet is not recommended.

This cookbook offers recipes to help you with incorporating keto foods that feel a little more special over the holidays. Explaining the fundamentals of a ketogenic diet is beyond the scope of this book, and we refer you to the website http://DietDoctor.com for excellent resources if you are just starting or would like to build your knowledge on ketogenic diets and nutritional ketosis.

Macronutrient Tracking

We've included macronutrient (macro) counts at the end of each recipe for easy tracking of protein, fats, and carbohydrates. We have broken carbohydrates (carbs) down even further into total and net carbs (total carbs minus the fiber content, as we don't digest fiber) as people like to use both, one or the other. Some lipedema ladies are happy to stick to 50 g total carbs (approximately 20 g net carbs) to be in ketosis, and others prefer to limit their carb intake to 20 g total for additional health benefits - this is totally up to you and your health goals.

Macro amounts have been calculated using Cronometer. Remember to increase or decrease the macros if having less or more of the serving size suggestion.

Nutritional ketosis is not about calorie restriction, it is about carbohydrate restriction, and therefore we haven't included calorie counts. Keto foods are naturally filling and satisfying. Being in ketosis acts as a natural appetite suppressant once fully fat adapted (when your body is more efficient at burning fat for energy), so people tend to find they need to eat fewer calories over time. 'Eat only when hungry, stop eating when comfortably full' is a guideline we encourage when following a keto lifestyle.

Food Allergy versus Food Intolerance

This book does not cater for people with food allergies. A food allergy is an immune response and can involve the digestive and respiratory systems, and can have severe and immediate reactions such as hives, digestive problems, swollen airways, blood in the stool, a drop in blood pressure and anaphylaxis. An allergic response can be life-threatening. Common food allergies are to peanuts, tree nuts, sesame seeds, milk, eggs, shellfish and fish, soy, wheat and lupin.

A food intolerance involves the digestive system and can also affect the respiratory tract, the nervous system and the skin. An intolerance can cause inflammation, swelling, pain, fatigue, abdominal pain and bloating after eating, diarrhea, constipation, reflux, heartburn, hives, face swelling, sinusitis, migraines, heart palpitations, joint pain, intestinal permeability, dermatitis, wheezing, coughing, asthma, nasal congestion and nasal polyps, mood and behavioral change, and more. Professional health advice should be sought to determine if you have a food allergy or food intolerance, and you will need to refer to recipe books that specifically cater to food allergies.

There are many food intolerances that we have not been able to cover in this book, such as salicylates, lectins, histamine, sulfites, amines, additives, preservatives, and more. We recommend seeking the help of a nutritionist to help you identify potential food intolerances.

Food Intolerances

Food intolerances are quite common for lipedema ladies, so each recipe is noted as either dairy-free, egg-free, nut-free, gluten-free, nightshade free and vegetarian (including lacto/ovo/pescatarian) or lists alternative options where applicable:

Gluten free I Egg free I Nut free I Dairy free
Nightshade free I Lacto/Ovo/Vegetarian/Pescatarian

Uniquely, we have explicitly catered for nightshade intolerance. It's not uncommon for women with lipedema, and other conditions such as autoimmune disease, for example, to be intolerant to the nightshade family which include (but are not limited to) bell peppers/capsicums, potatoes (potato starch is used in some grated cheese and other processed foods), aubergine/eggplant, tomatoes, chilies, cayenne pepper, red pepper flakes, paprika (often hidden in anything labeled 'spices'). We have tailored the recipes to either remove or replace nightshade ingredients.

FODMAPs (fermentable fructans, oligosaccharides, disaccharides, monosaccharides, and polyols) is a form of carbohydrate malabsorption, and these are found in many foods such as fructose in fruit, vegetables and grains, and lactose in milk. Determining if digestive upset is caused by FODMAPs is unfortunately outside of the scope of this recipe book.

You can find further information on FODMAPs at https://www.monashfodmap.com/. A low FODMAP diet is an elimination type diet. It is not intended as a long-term dietary approach, and it is best to seek the help of a Nutritionist to help you to determine if this is something you need to explore.

A food intolerance is often dose dependent, meaning you may be able to tolerate small amounts without a response. A cumulative effect can mean that once you go over your body's limit you then experience symptoms.

Emulsifiers

Processed and packaged foods often contain emulsifiers, which are used to combine, smooth, and thicken ingredients that don't normally mix well, such as oil and lemon juice. Emulsifiers can also act as anti-nutrients by blocking the absorption of minerals such as calcium.

Additionally, people with non-celiac gluten sensitivity or celiac disease, or people who have compromised digestive health, gastrointestinal conditions or autoimmune disease may be very sensitive to emulsifiers, as these additives are known to increase gastrointestinal inflammation. Some act as laxatives. They can disrupt our gut microbiome and are thought to damage the intestinal barrier function in some people.

We recommend you always check the ingredient list for all dairy products, non-dairy milk products such as coconut and almond milk, and other packaged food products. Common emulsifiers to avoid are wheat starch, wheat barley or rye based modified food starch, guar gum, locust bean gum, carrageenan, xanthan gum and cellulose gum.

Gluten

For people with non-celiac gluten sensitivity or celiac disease, always check packaged food ingredient labels and allergen warnings. Some food ingredients differ from brand to brand and country of manufacture. For example, some cheeses do not contain gluten as a whole product, however, may contain gluten additives when pre-grated or processed. Low salt, low fat and no fat dairy can contain gluten, however we always promote full fat dairy products as the carbohydrate count is lower and they are more satisfying. Blue cheese can potentially contain gluten if the mold cultures are grown on wheat or rye bread. You also need to avoid hydrolyzed vegetable and hydrolyzed plant proteins, so always check the ingredient label and allergen lists.

Additives in dairy such as wheat starch and modified food starch made from wheat or barley (rarely rye) may contain gluten and can be found in products such as cottage cheese. If vinegar is an ingredient always check to ensure it's not malt vinegar, which is made from barley and therefore contains gluten (also avoid malt flavouring). Bacon typically doesn't contain gluten; however cross-contamination can occur with any food if manufacturing takes place in a shared facility or with shared equipment, and this can be the case for many foods labelled as gluten-free and not guaranteed gluten-free.

Additional sources of hidden gluten include powdered cellulose, maltodextrin, artificial and natural flavors, fillers and spice mixes.

Individual herbs and spices are not always gluten-free. They can contain a non-gluten anti- caking agent such as silicon dioxide, sodium aluminium silica or calcium silicate. Also, there have been instances where spices have had wheat flour or wheat starch added to increase product volume. Cross-contamination with gluten is also a possibility with herbs and spices, depending on the manufacturer and their methods, as described above. This may not be as much of an issue with non-celiac gluten sensitivity as it is with celiac disease, however everyone reacts differently.

If you have celiac disease, there are additional food items which are not contained in this book, and consumer products such as personal hygiene products, that also contain gluten. Even trace elements of gluten ingested or used on the skin can be harmful, however that is outside of the scope of this recipe book.

Dairy

Dairy can cause insulin to spike, and raised insulin suppresses ketones and impedes weight loss. A1 beta-casein, a protein found in dairy can activate the inflammatory pathway and many women with lipedema and lipo-lymphedema find dairy can increase swelling. The degree to which this causes a problem depends on your tolerance of dairy proteins. In these instances, we recommend you speak with a health professional trained in ketogenic diets to help you individualize your intake and recommend alternative nutrient sources if required, such as calcium. People with lactose intolerance lack the enzyme lactase, which is required to digest the dairy sugar lactose, and is dose dependent.

Another, less well-known type of dairy intolerance involves the proteins found in dairy; whey and/or casein. This type of intolerance can cause digestive upset, increased swelling and other symptoms. Professional advice should be sought to differentiate this response from a food allergy if symptoms go beyond the digestive system and involve the respiratory system and swelling of any kind including the throat or face.

For people with a food intolerance, substituting dairy products made with A1 milk for products made with A2 milk can, in some instances, be better tolerated. A2 products are usually found in goat and sheep dairy, as well as dairy produced from Southern European cows in Switzerland, France, Italy and Spain. Few products certify they only contain A1 dairy if you are particularly sensitive, however there are brands that do.

Sugar and Flour Substitutes

Sweeteners and flour replacements such as almond flour are not typically recommended for lipedema ladies due to their effect on spiking insulin, sweet cravings, food intolerances, digestive upset, dysbiosis, swelling, and joint pain for some women.

Liquid stevia is preferred, although it doesn't always suit a recipe such as the pecan torte in this book, which requires 'Gentle Sweet' (a mixture of erythritol, xylitol and stevia) for structural integrity. Try to avoid granulated stevia unless you know it is pure, as it often contains sugar, maltodextrin or artificial sweeteners.

Sugar alcohols contain FODMAPs (see food intolerance section) and some people with this form of carbohydrate malabsorption are only able to tolerate very small amounts of the foods they are contained in, if at all. Sugar alcohols such as xylitol do have carbohydrates, some of which we digest and some we don't, so you can take approximately 50% off the total sugar alcohol amount from the total carb amount to give you a net carb figure. Erythritol does not count towards carbohydrates as it isn't digested.

Adding sweeteners and flour replacements occasionally for holiday dishes can be better than their high carbohydrate alternatives which will likely kick you out of ketosis and potentially increase symptoms that have reduced or disappeared while in ketosis.

Aim to keep serving sizes small when using sweeteners and alternative flours.

Mindful Eating

Decadent foods, especially ones prepared with sweeteners, can be challenging for some people to not overeat. Here we encourage 'mindful eating', a practice whereby you refocus your thoughts by bringing them back into the moment, by doing something that will help you to feel calm and centered before eating. It can also help to slow down how fast you eat and encourage better digestion.

An exercise to try: before your next meal, sit down (in a quiet place and close your eyes) and concentrate on your breathing for one minute, taking slow, deep breaths. If you feel lightheaded then stop, and gradually build up to one minute. Take note of how you feel before and after the deep breathing. Repeat when needed for a calm approach to eating.

Happy Holidays!

Megan

Megan Pfeffer, BHSc
Clinical Nutritionist
Specialist in Therapeutic Nutrition
megan@lipedema-simplified.org

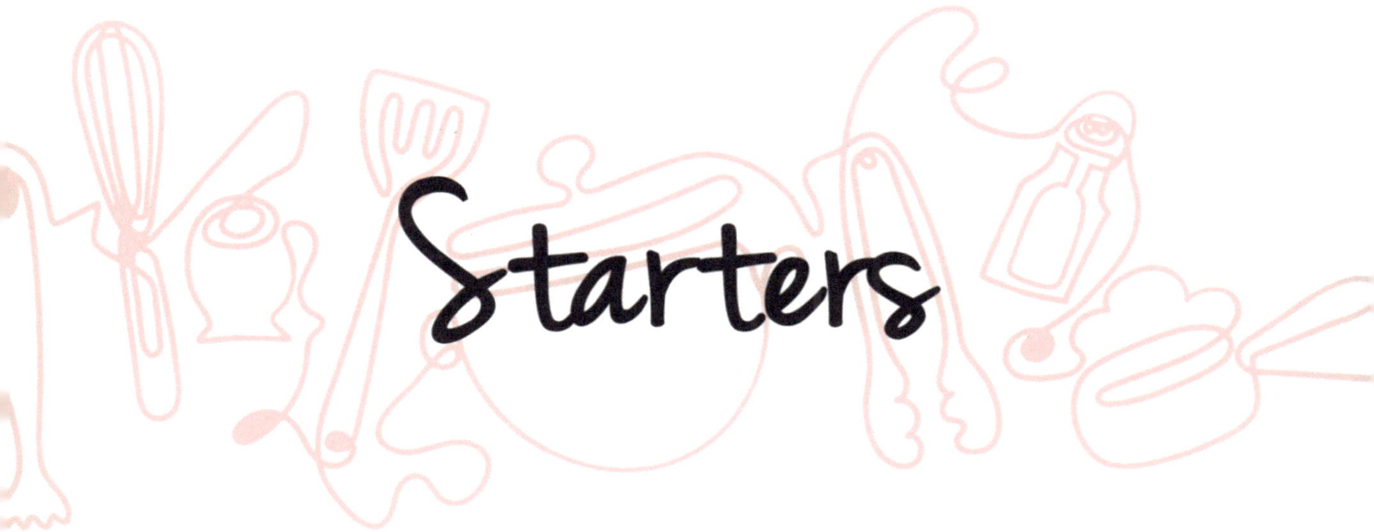

Starters

"For me, when I handle vegetables, there is something very precious about them and I want to bring out the best in them. That's cutting things, tasting things and sensing things closely enough to know what I like, what I don't like, and how to honor the sincerity and integrity of the vegetable." ~Edward Espe Brown

Starters

Assorted Charcuterie Board

Catherine & Mende

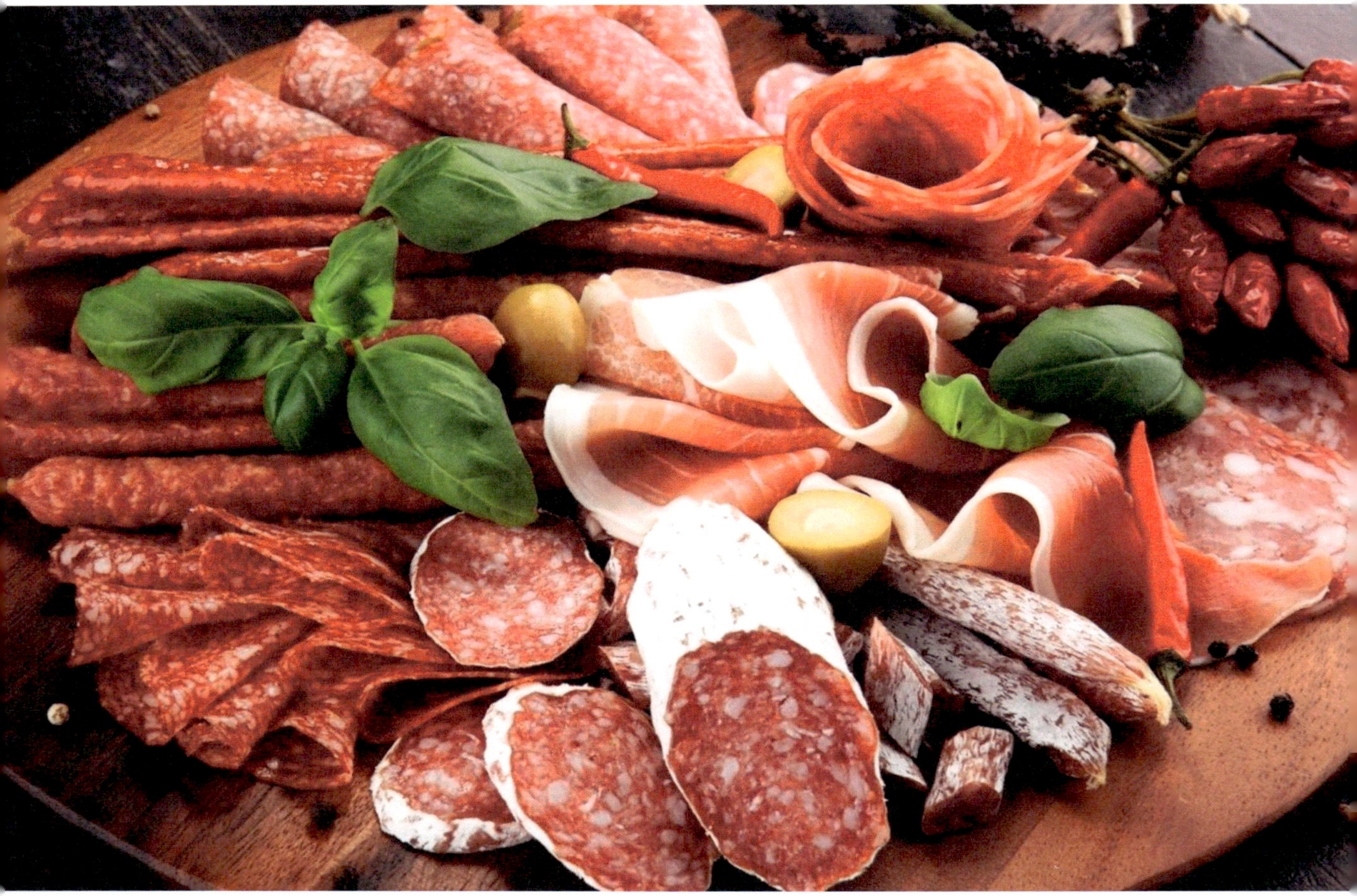

Servings: 10

Ingredients:

15 oz. ǀ 450 g of your favorite meats, salami*, pepperoni* and prosciutto are pictured. You can also use ham, chicken or sausages**

15 oz. ǀ 450 g of your favorite cheeses, such as brie and

7 ½ oz. ǀ 225 g assorted olives in brine

7 ½ oz. ǀ 225 g pickles (no sugar) 7 ½ oz. ǀ 225 g raw vegetables*

3.5 oz. ǀ 100 g celery

3.5 oz. ǀ 100 g herbed cream cheese

You can also serve with one of the dips, seed crackers or avocado crackers (see recipes) - these are not included in the macro count.

Method:

1. Arrange everything on a board and serve chilled.

* If nightshade intolerant, omit bell peppers/capsicums, tomatoes, chilli, salami & pepperoni, check if sausages contain 'spices', chilli or cayenne pepper.

**Most sausages contain wheat, and many contain eggs and/or milk. Also check the ingredient list for nightshades such as potato starch, paprika, chilli and cayenne pepper.

* If nightshade intolerant, omit bell peppers/capsicums, tomatoes, chilli, salami & pepperoni, check if sausages contain 'spices', chilli or cayenne pepper.

**Most sausages contain wheat, and many contain eggs and/or milk. Also check the ingredient list for nightshades such as potato starch, paprika, chilli and cayenne pepper.

Egg free option | Nut free | Dairy free option | Nightshade free option

Serving size	Protein	Fat	Total Carbs	Net Carbs
5.9 oz 168 g	20.3 g	32.8 g	5.2 g	3.5 g

Caprese Salad

Mende

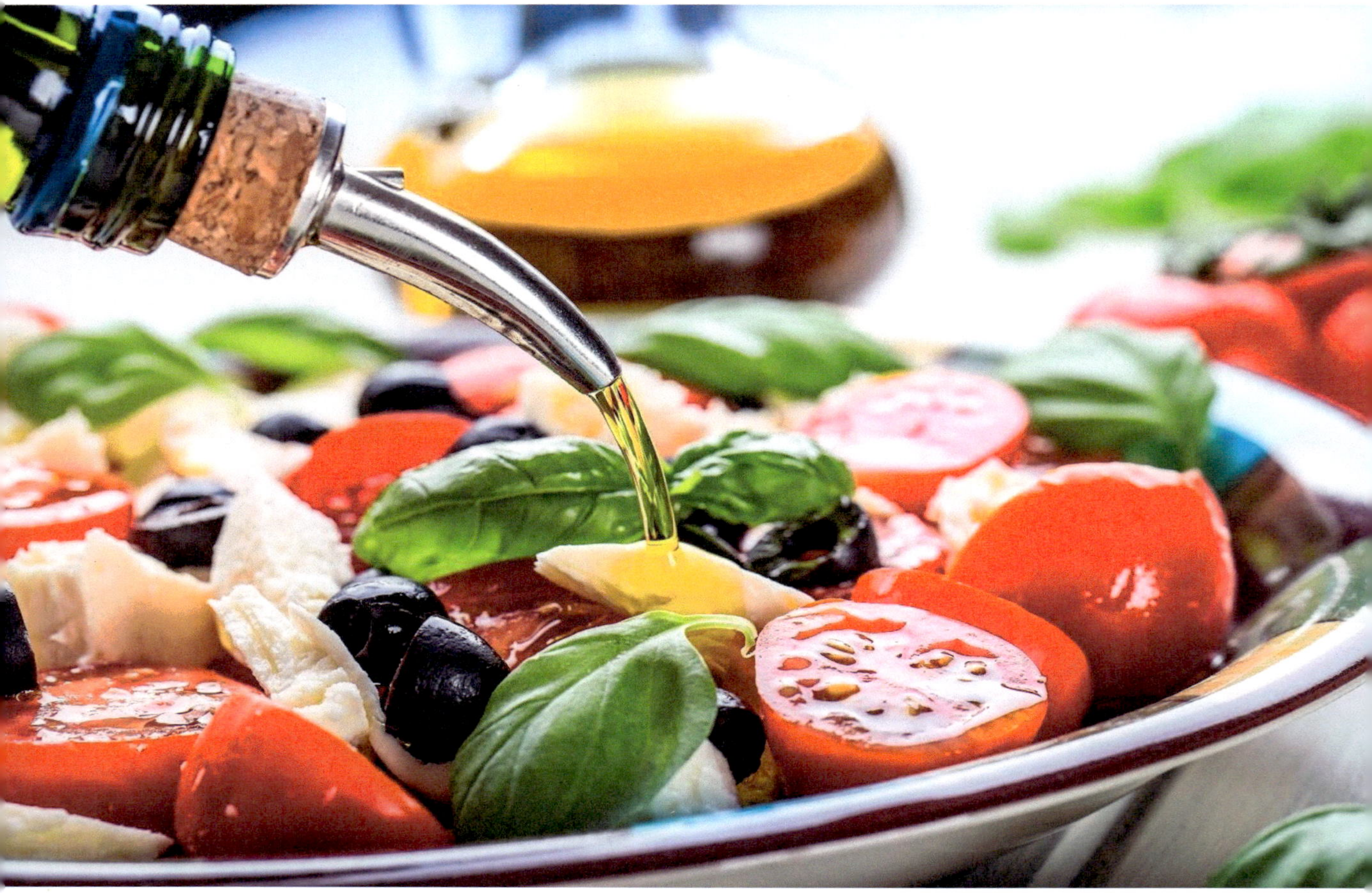

Servings: 8

Ingredients:

1 lb l450 g mozzarella (fresh) pearls or slices*
1 lb l450 g grape or cherry tomatoes**
1 bunch fresh basil – 20-30 leaves
½ cup extra virgin olive oil
¼ cup red wine vinegar Salt and pepper to taste
½ cup l90 g olives (optional) - *my favorites are kalamata olives*

Method:

1. Drain mozzarella. If using slices, cut each slice into quarters.
2. Cut tomatoes in half.
3. Clean, wash and dry basil.
4. To chiffonade basil, stack the leaves, roll tightly, slice the roll into ribbons.
5. Combine tomatoes, basil and mozzarella in a serving bowl.
6. Combine olive oil, vinegar, salt and pepper to taste in a jar with a lid.
7. Shake the jar to combine then drizzle over the salad.
8. Garnish with olives (optional, included in the macro count).

* If dairy intolerant replace mozzarella with ripe avocado.
** If nightshade intolerant replace tomatoes with cucumbers.

Gluten free I Egg free I Nut free I Dairy free option Nightshade free option I Vegetarian

Serving size	Protein	Fat	Total Carbs	Net Carbs
5oz/150g	12.8 g	30.5 g	4.5 g	2.2 g

Christmas Eve Salad

Raeann

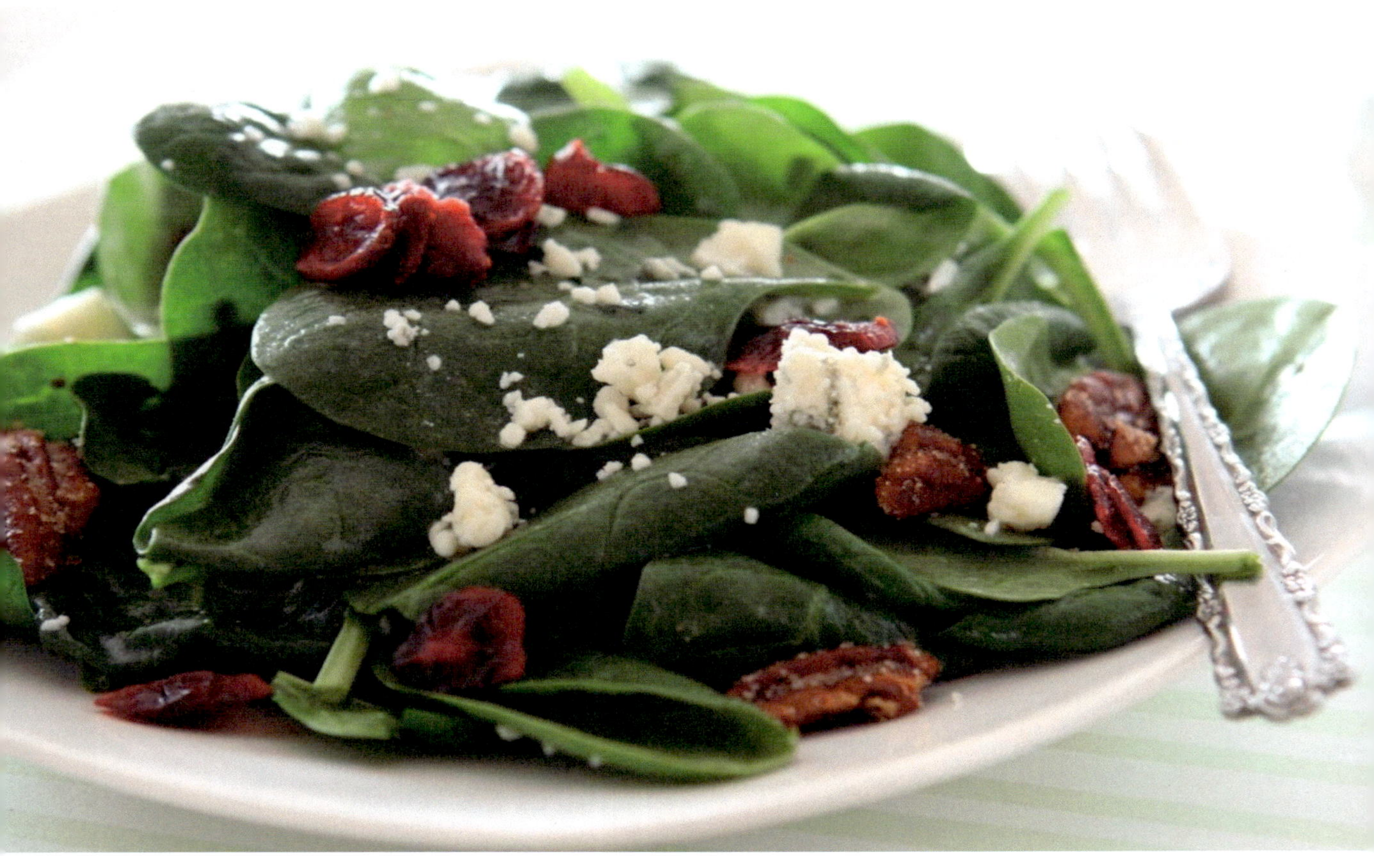

Servings: 10

Ingredients:

6 cups raw spinach, torn
1 cup | 136 g raw beetroot, peeled & cut into cubes
1/2 cup raw pecans, coarsely chopped*
4 oz | 113 g fresh goat cheese, like Chèvre
1/4 cup extra virgin olive oil
3 tablespoons balsamic vinegar
1/4 teaspoon pumpkin pie spice**, or to taste
3 dashes | 3 g natural salt, or to taste
2 dashes | 2 g pepper, or to taste

Method:

1. Pre-heat oven to 350°F/175°C.
2. Spread pecans in a single layer on a roasting pan and toast until lightly browned (about 6-8 minutes – check frequently so you don't burn them).
3. Take the pecans out of your roasting pan, salt and set aside.
4. Increase oven temperature to 425°F/200°C.
5. Add the beets into the pan. Stir in the olive oil and pumpkin pie spice.
6. Roast at 425°F/200°C for 10 minutes or until done and beets can be easily pierced..
7. While the beet mixture is roasting, wash, drain and tear spinach into a salad bowl. Crumble goat cheese over the top.
8. Remove roasting pan from the oven. Add balsamic vinegar, salt and pepper to taste and stir to create a warm vinaigrette in the roasting pan.
9. Scrape roasted beet mixture from roasting pan onto spinach and crumbled goat cheese in the salad bowl. Top with toasted pecans and serve immediately with a slice of Tourtiere (see recipe).

*Omit pecans for nut free.

** Check for gluten free.

Gluten free option | Egg free | Nut free option | Nightshade free | Lacto Vegetarian

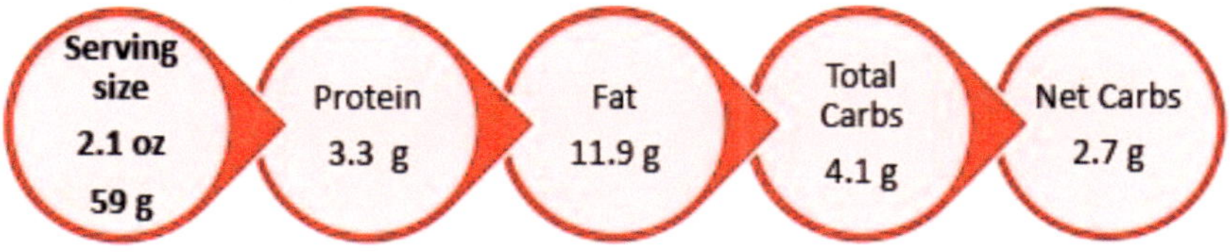

Chopped Liver

Carol

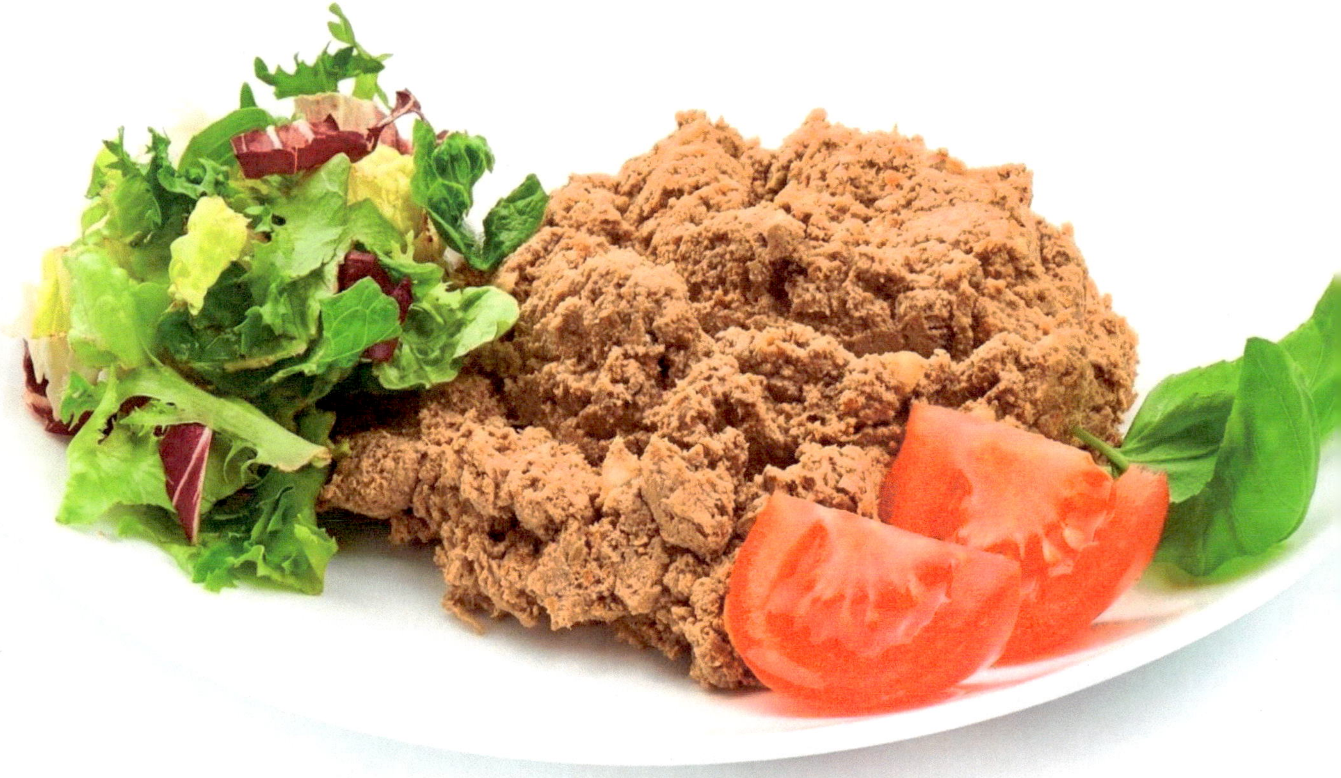

Servings: 10 (as a starter)

Good for any occasion. Even those who dislike liver often love this recipe!

Ingredients:

1 lb | 450 g chicken livers, preferably organic
2 medium brown or white onions, diced
2 eggs, hard boiled plus one extra hard-cooked yolk
½ teaspoon salt
2 tablespoons rendered chicken fat, or your preferred tasteless fat
Lettuce, enough to cover your serving plate

Method:

1. Fry the liver and onions in chicken fat until livers are no longer pink inside. Refrigerate to cool.
2. Put all ingredients through a meat grinder. Add salt to taste. Add more rendered fat to create a pasty texture so that the mixture can be spread with a knife. Place into a container and seal, then refrigerate for a minimum of 1 hour.
3. Spoon the cold mixture onto a bed of lettuce arranged on your serving plate.
4. Using a fork, break up the extra yolk and sprinkle on top of the liver.
5. If not avoiding nightshades, you can sprinkle some paprika on top of the yolk.

TIP: Serve on seed crackers or avocado crackers (see recipes) - these are not included in the macro or serving size counts. If desired, use as a roll-up with lettuce, or spread on cucumber slices or celery.

Gluten free | Nut free | Dairy free | Nightshade free option

Serving size	Protein	Fat	Total Carbs	Net Carbs
3.2 oz 90g	12.7 g	8.1 g	2.9 g	2.4 g

Crackers with Avocado

Mende

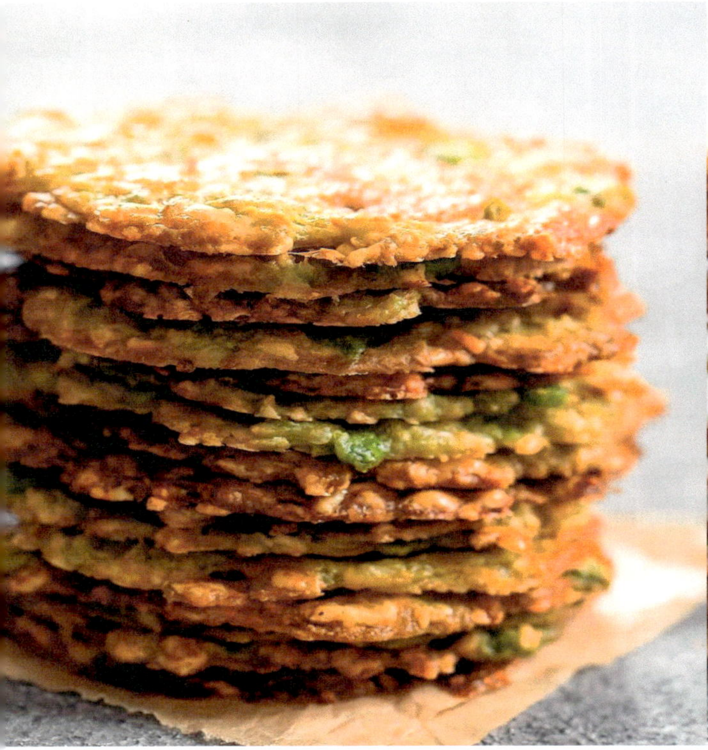

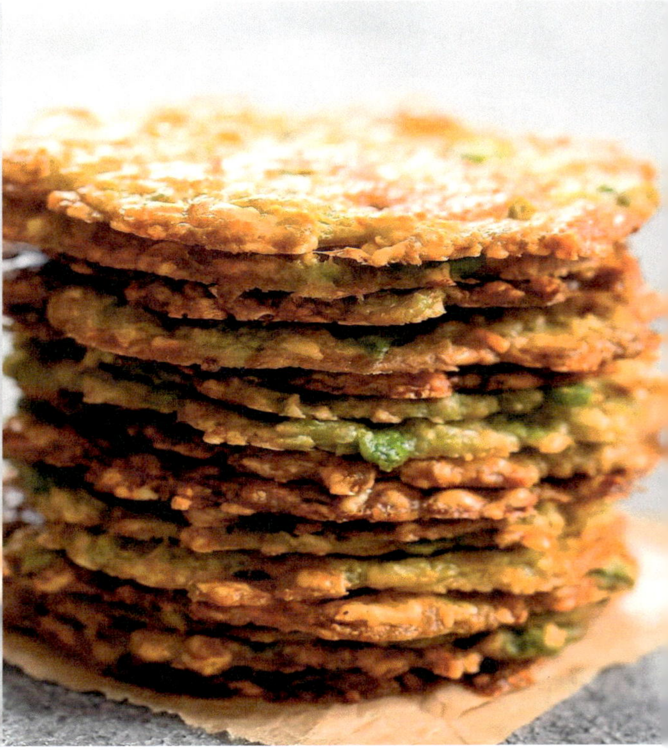

Servings: 8

Ingredients:

1 ½ avocados, peeled and mashed
1 ¼ cups parmesan cheese*, grated
¼ teaspoon onion powder*
¼ teaspoon garlic powder*
Dash cayenne pepper*

Method:

1. Preheat oven to 300 °F/150 °C.
2. Mix all ingredients together with a spoon and roll out between two sheets of parchment paper.
3. Remove top sheet of paper and score with a pastry cutter, pizza cutter, or a knife.
4. Bake for approx. 15 minutes or until lightly browned. Cool slightly.
5. Cut and separate pieces. Turn oven to warm and continue to bake until pieces are dry and crispy.

*Check for gluten free herbs. Check gluten and nightshade (potato starch) free if pre-grated parmesan. Omit cayenne pepper if nightshade intolerant.

Egg free | Nut free | Nightshade free | Vegetarian

Serving size	Protein	Fat	Total Carbs	Net Carbs
1.9oz/54g	9.9 g	9.9 g	5.5 g	2.9 g

Crackers with Seeds

Catherine

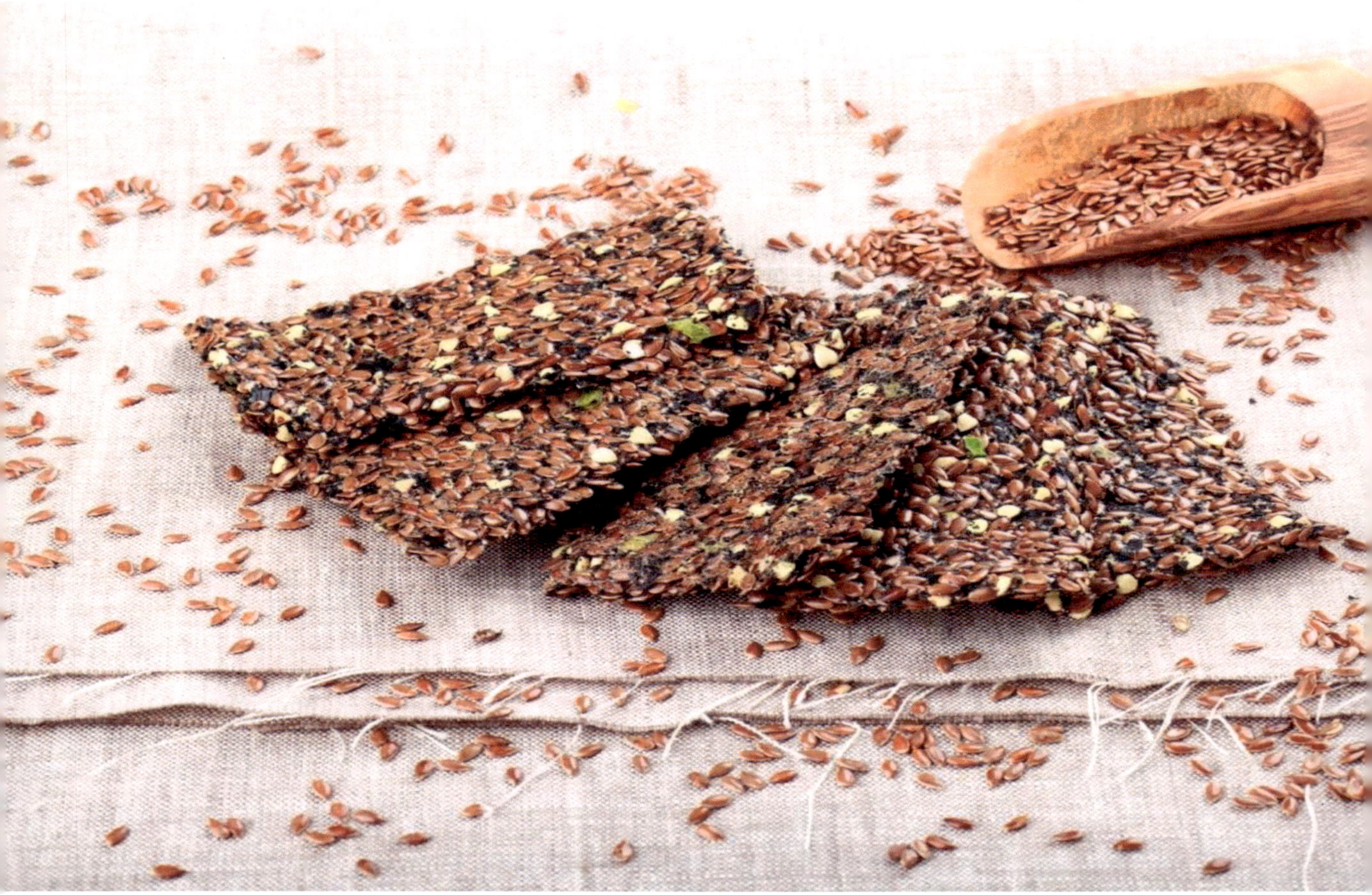

Servings: 32 (2 crackers per serving)

Ingredients:

2 cups brown or golden or combination flax seeds*

1 cup sesame seeds*

½ cup pumpkin seeds*

½ cup sunflower seeds*

½ cup chia seeds*

6-8 cups of water

Note: The seeds need to soak for 1-2 hours prior to baking

Variations:

Savory: add salt, onion powder, herbs - add to taste

Sweet: add cinnamon, pumpkin pie spices, flavorings such as vanilla or almond

Note: variations not included in macro count.

Method:

1. Combine flax and sesame seeds in a big bowl and add 8 cups of water.
2. Let set for 1-2 hours, stirring occasionally.
3. The seeds absorb the water and become batter-like.
4. Slowly sprinkle chia seeds over the mixture, stirring well.
5. Chia seeds absorb water quickly so you might need to add in additional water - keep the batter a similar consistency to pancake batter (or more dense depending on how you like your crackers).
6. Add in pumpkin seeds and sunflower seeds stirring well.
7. Line cookie sheets with parchment paper.
8. Spoon mixture and spread evenly then score into squares or rectangles - this recipe makes 32 crackers.
9. Bake at 175 °F/80 °C for several hours or until done (I bake mine overnight on the lowest setting).
10. Let cool and break into cracker sizes.
11. Store in airtight container lined with parchment paper.
12. Will stay fresh for quite a while - a month or two.

*Check allergen list for gluten.

Gluten free option | Egg free | Nut free |
Dairy free | Nightshade free | Vegetarian

Serving size	Protein	Fat	Total Carbs	Net Carbs
0.7 oz 21 g	4.8 g	8 g	5.1 g	3.8 g

Happy Kwanzaa

good things happen around a table

Herbed Sour Cream Dip

Mende

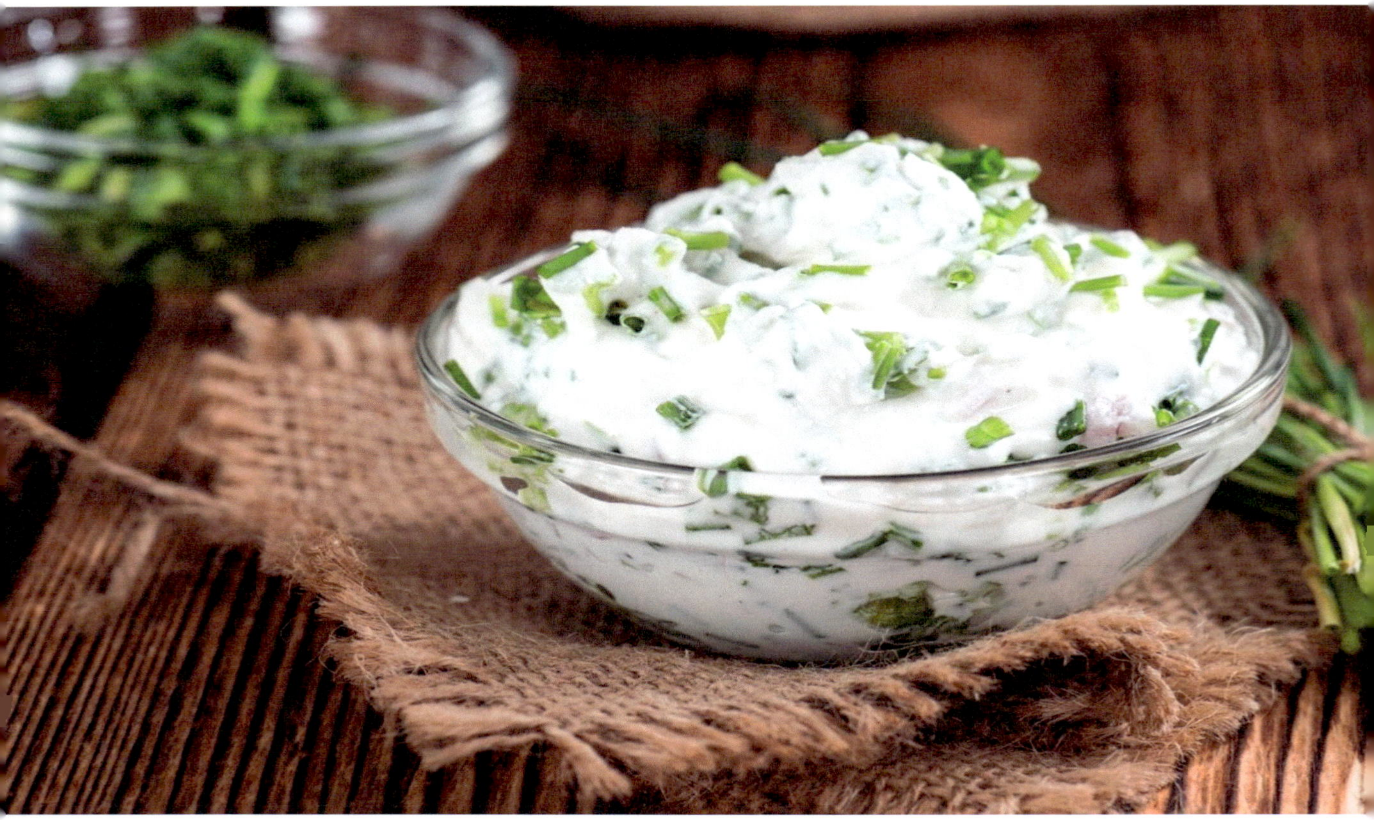

Servings: 8

Ingredients:

16 oz | 450 g sour cream
1 cup extra virgin olive oil mayo or avocado oil mayo (Primal Kitchens brand is widely available)
¼ teaspoon salt
Pinch of coarsely ground black pepper

1 teaspoon dried oregano** 1 teaspoon dried parsley**
1 teaspoon dried dill weed**
¼ teaspoon onion powder **
¼ teaspoon garlic powder**

Note: Check allergen warning for gluten. Alter herbs and spices to your taste. Mayo used in macro count.

Method:

1. Combine all ingredients.
2. Serve with pork rinds (omit if vegetarian) and/or raw vegetables (not included in the recipe macro count).

*Check allergen list for gluten.

Gluten free option | Nut free | Nightshade free | Lacto Vegetarian

Serving size	Protein	Fat	Total Carbs	Net Carbs
3 oz 86 g	1.5 g	33.9 g	2.9 g	2.8 g

New Year's Eve Cheeseball

Mende

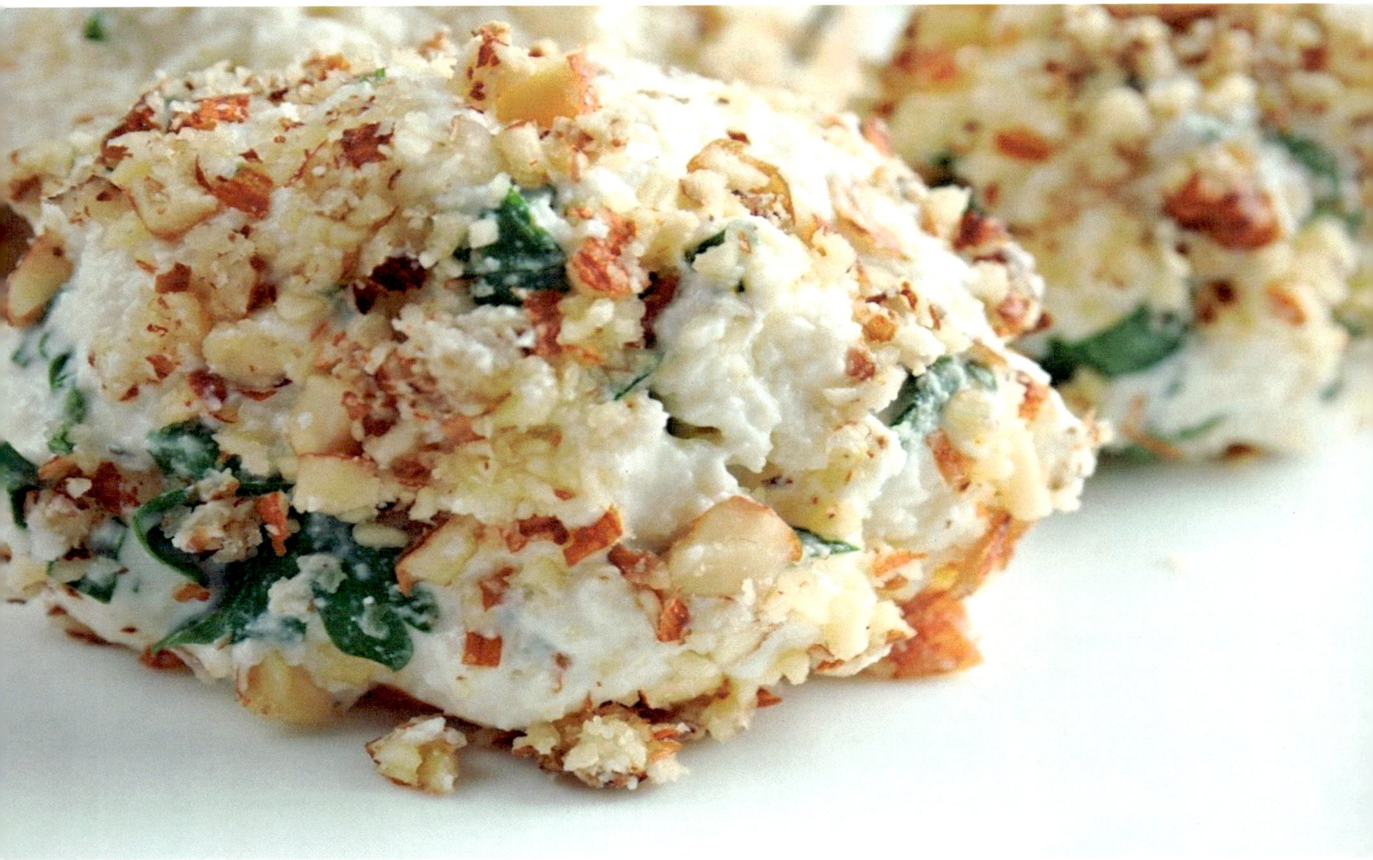

Servings: 12

This is even better when made 24 hours in advance.

Ingredients:

1 pound | 450 g cream cheese, softened
1 cup Primal Kitchens' mayo
2 tablespoon mustard
½ teaspoon garlic powder
1 teaspoon worcestershire sauce
1 x 2.25 oz. jar | 65 g Armour dried beef, chopped OR substitute 2 oz| 56 g pastrami
1 bunch green onions, minced
2 cups shredded cheese, *sharp cheddar is my favorite*
Salt and black pepper, to taste

Additional Options:

1 cup cooked baby shrimp or ½ cup chopped smoked salmon (replacing the beef with shrimp or salmon makes a pescaterian version).
Leave out meat and fish for a vegetarian version.

Serve with celery sticks, cheese crisps, avocado or seed crackers, or pork rinds (not included in macro count).

Method:

1. Mix softened cream cheese with mayonnaise. Beat until smooth.
2. Stir in seasonings, beef, onions and shredded cheese.
3. Shape into a ball or wreath, or mound into a serving bowl.
4. Chill thoroughly before serving.

Nut free | Pescatarian option

Serving size	Protein	Fat	Total Carbs	Net Carbs
2.8 oz 81 g	6.3 g	31.6 g	3.4 g	3.2 g

Pumpkin Soup

Mende

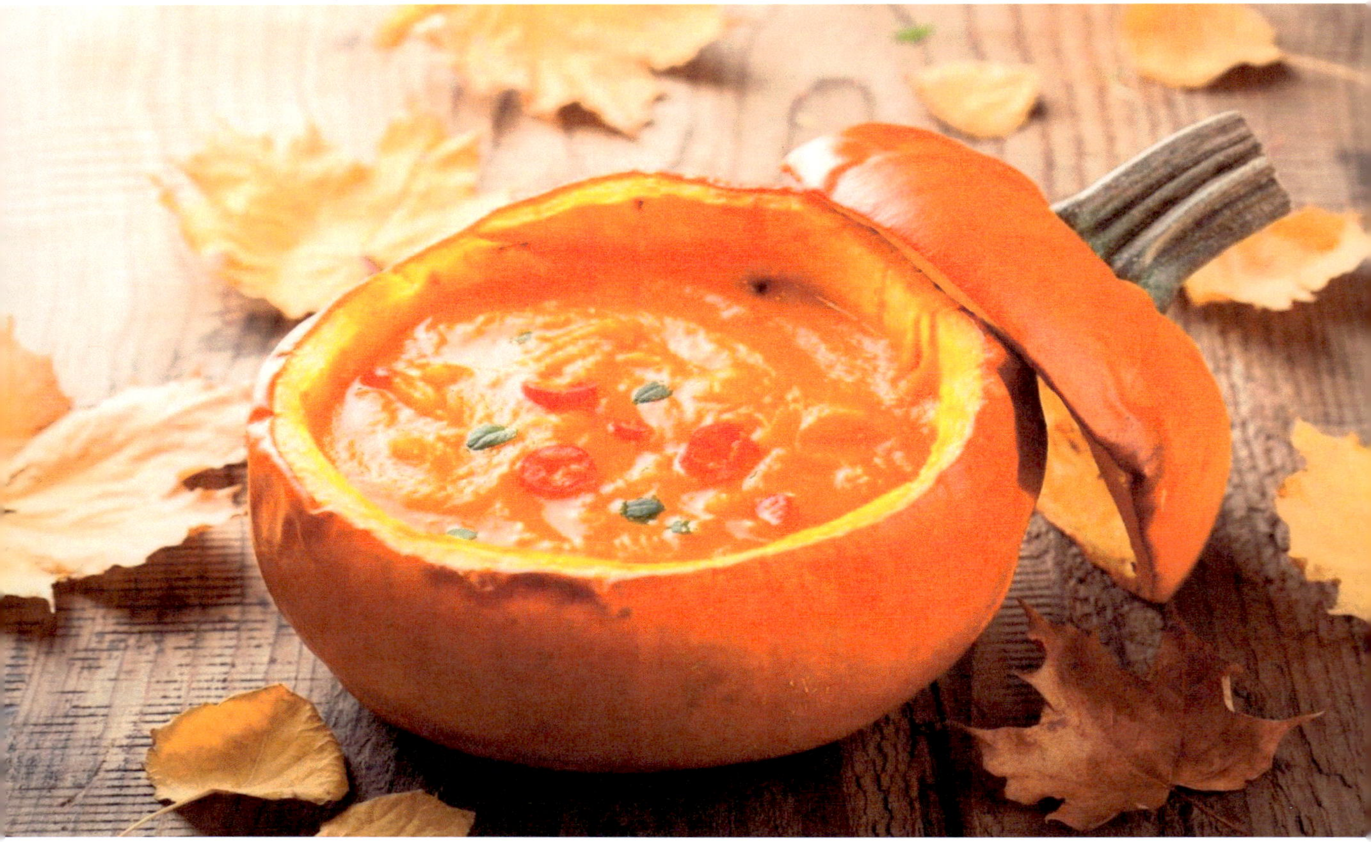

Servings: 6

Ingredients:

1 x 15 oz can | 425 g pumpkin puree (not pumpkin pie filling)
3 ½ cups homemade or store-bought chicken stock or store-bought chicken broth*
1 teaspoon salt, or to taste
½ teaspoon ground white pepper
½ teaspoon onion powder**
½ teaspoon poultry seasoning or rubbed sage**
¼ teaspoon freshly grated nutmeg
1 cup heavy cream***

To Serve:

¼ cup sour cream or creme fraiche
2 tablespoon chopped parsley or a few additional grates of nutmeg

Note: Macro count based on using chicken broth and sour cream to serve.

Method:

1. Add the pumpkin puree, chicken broth, salt, pepper, onion powder, poultry seasoning and nutmeg to a medium saucepan. Stir to combine.
2. Bring the mixture to a boil, then reduce heat and simmer for about 10 minutes, to give the flavors time to meld.
3. Remove from the heat, and add the heavy cream.
4. If desired, garnish with sour cream or creme fraiche, parsley or nutmeg.

* Check allergen warning for gluten, check for spices if nightshade intolerant, replace with vegetable stock for vegetarian option
** Check allergen warning for gluten.
*** Check for emulsifiers.

Gluten free option | Egg free | Nut free | Nightshade free option | LactoVegetarian

Serving size	Protein	Fat	Total Carbs	Net Carbs
13.8 oz 393 g	7.6 g	27.3 g	12.4 g	9.6 g

Spinach Artichoke Dip

Mende

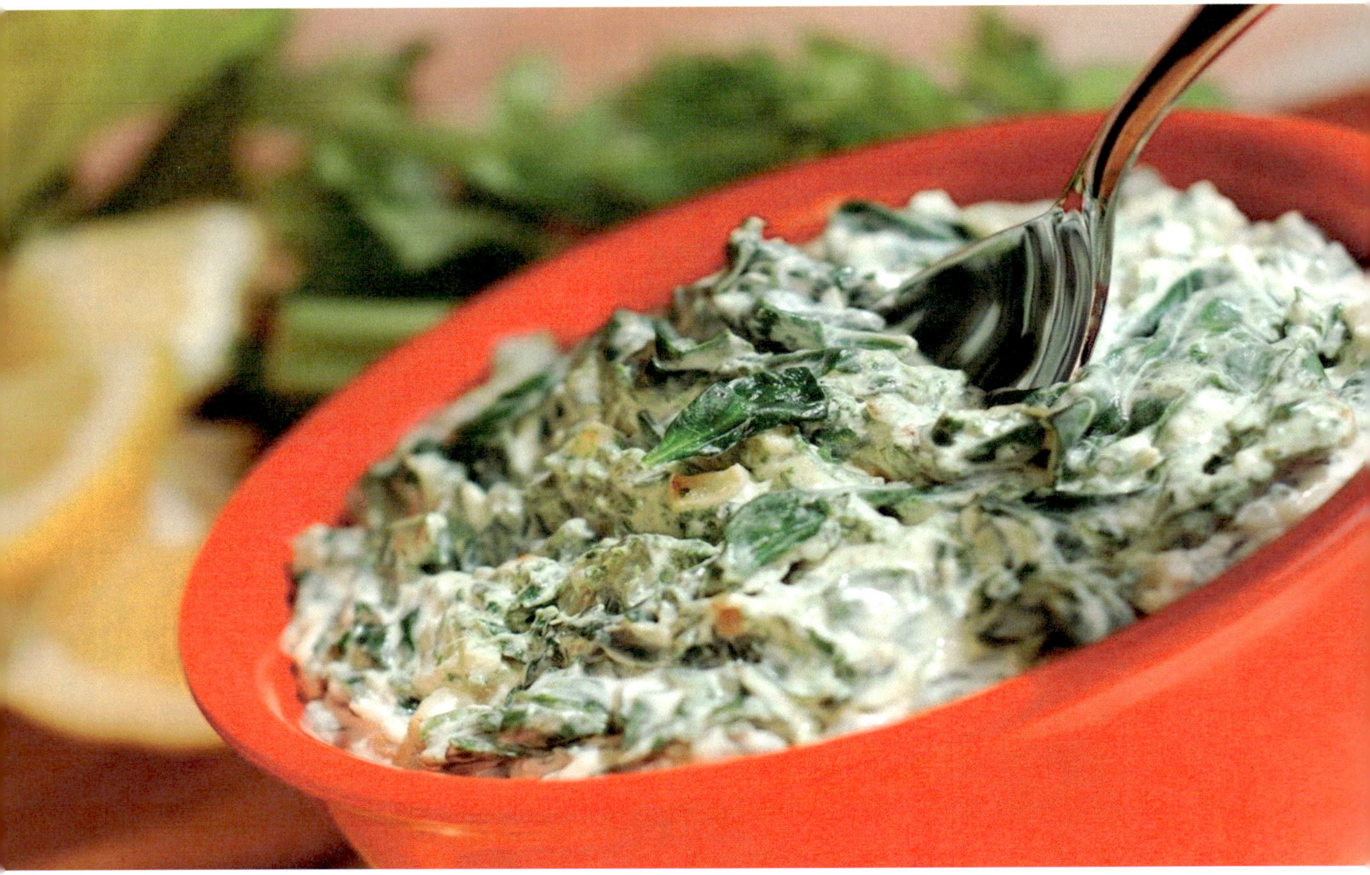

Servings: 8

Ingredients:

4 oz | 120 g frozen spinach, thawed
8 oz | 250 g block cream cheese, at room temp
6 oz | 170 g bottled or canned artichoke hearts in brine, finely chopped
½ cup shredded mozzarella cheese*
¼ cup finely grated parmesan cheese*
1 tablespoon minced garlic
Salt to taste

Method:

1. Preheat oven to 400° F/200° C.
2. Squeeze & discard all excess liquid from the spinach.
3. In a medium-sized bowl, combine the spinach, cream cheese, artichokes, mozzarella, parmesan and garlic; mix well to combine (use your hands if necessary).
4. Place in a baking dish and bake until hot and bubbly.
5. Serve with pork rinds (omit if vegetarian) or fresh veggies for dipping.

*Check for potato starch if nightshade intolerant, and check allergen warning for gluten.

Gluten free option | Egg free | Nut free | Nightshade free option | Lacto Vegetarian

Serving size	Protein	Fat	Total Carbs	Net Carbs
2.7 oz 79 g	5.2 g	13.2 g	4.1 g	3.1 g

Eat, Drink & Be Merrily

Ketolicious

Main Dishes

"Carefully tasting what you put in your mouth is extremely important. By giving yourself over to the experience and by allowing yourself to actually find out what's in the experience, when you do that, you'll make wiser choices." ~Edward Espe Brown

Main Dishes

BBQ Ribs Oven Roasted

Mende

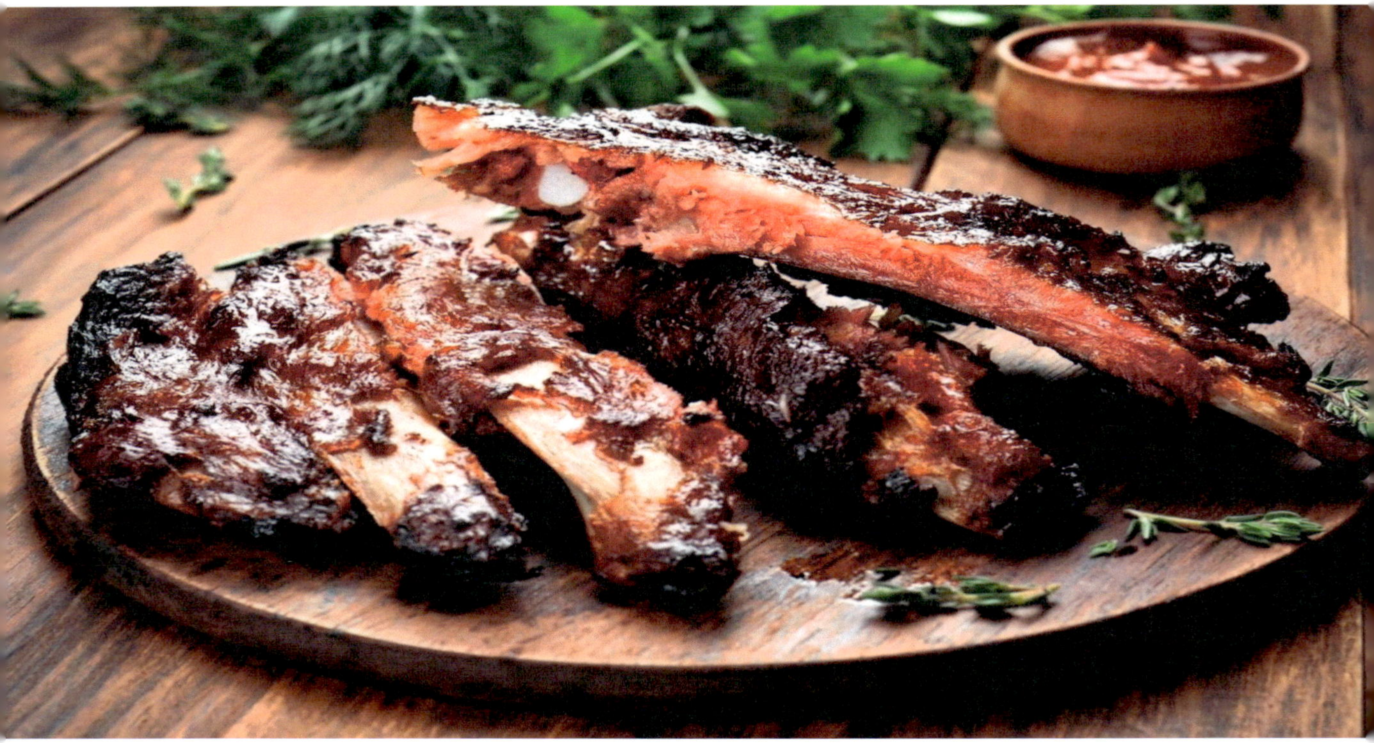

Servings: 4

Ingredients:

For the Ribs:

1 pound | 450 g country-style pork ribs or pork steak

¼ cup light extra virgin olive oil

½ teaspoon Wright's Hickory liquid smoke

Dry Rub:

1 teaspoon Salt
¼ teaspoon ground black pepper
1 teaspoon garlic powder
½ teaspoon smoked paprika
1 teaspoon Mrs. Dash original

For the Sauce:

1 cup salted chicken or beef broth
½ teaspoon garlic powder
¼ teaspoon onion powder
¼ teaspoon smoked paprika* (omit if nightshade intolerant)
¼ teaspoon allspice
¼ teaspoon black pepper or cayenne pepper* (omit cayenne if nightshade intolerant)
A few drops of liquid smoke.

Method for the ribs:

1. Preheat oven to 300° F/150° C.
2. In a large bowl, whisk together olive oil and liquid smoke. Toss the pork in this mixture to coat.
3. Remove pork to a plate and sprinkle both sides liberally with the spices listed above.
4. Prepare a large baking pan by wrapping with aluminum foil. Place ribs on foil-lined pan, leaving space in between each piece. Roast 1 ½ to 2 ½ hours in the oven until the meat is tender and nicely browned.

Method for the sauce:

1. Combine the above in a medium saucepan. Bring to a boil, stirring constantly.
2. Cook until reduced by half (takes only a few minutes).
3. Stir in 1/4 cup red wine vinegar or apple cider vinegar or plain white vinegar. Drizzle over the finished ribs or use as a dipping sauce.

* Omit Mrs Dash original and smoked paprika if nightshade intolerant.

Note: It may not be ideal to consume smoked foods such as liquid smoke too frequently due to carcinogenic polycyclic aromatic hydrocarbons.

Egg free | Nut free | Dairy free

Serving size	Protein	Fat	Total Carbs	Net Carbs
6.6 oz 188g	34 g	47.6 g	0.7 g	0.6 g

In cooking you've got to have a what-the-hell attitude.

~Julia Child

Beef Bourguignon Pot Roast

Mende

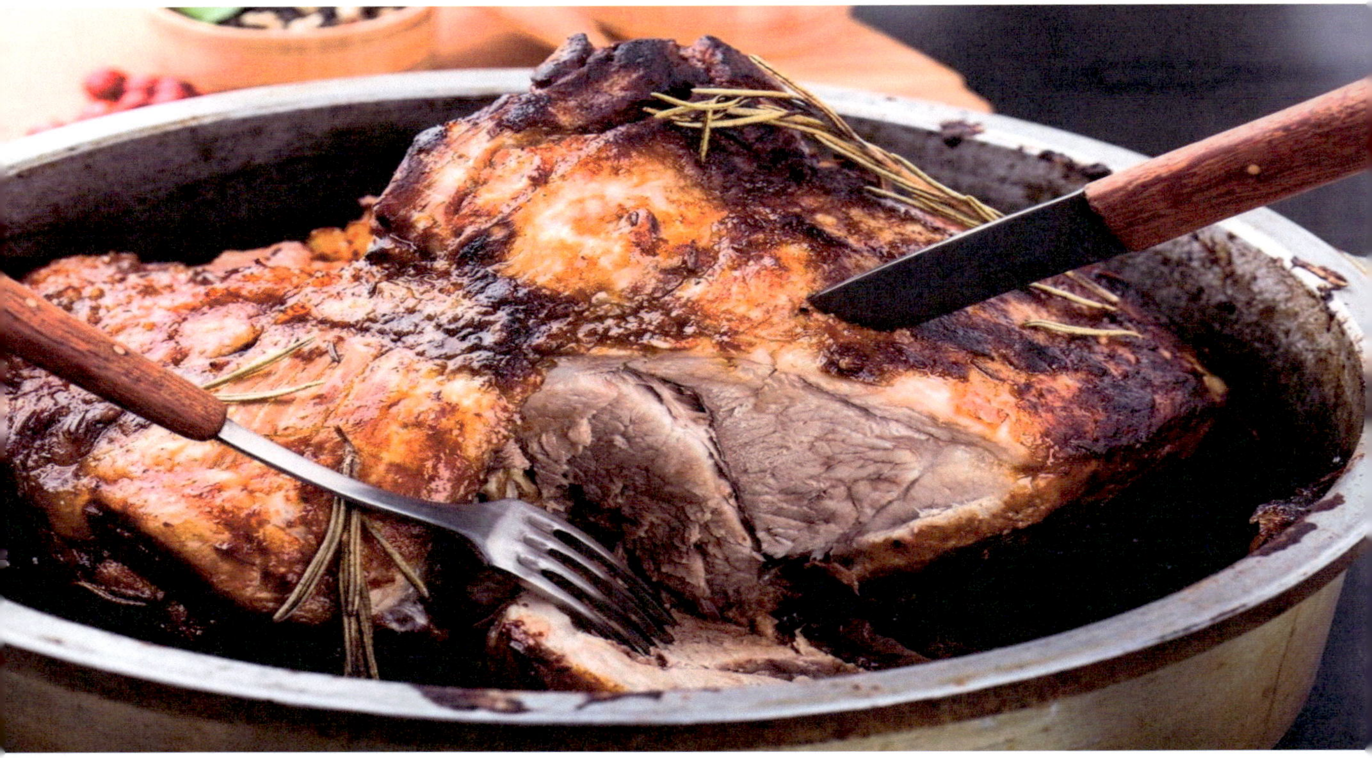

Servings: 12

Ingredients:

3 pounds I 1.6 kg chuck roast (or thereabouts)
Pink salt, Redmond's real salt or your favorite salt
3 ribs celery, thinly sliced
½ onion, thinly sliced
1 pinch crushed red pepper (use black pepper if nightshade intolerant)
3 cloves garlic, smashed and finely chopped
1 cup dry red wine
4 cups chicken stock*
3 bay leaves
1 fresh thyme bundle
2 cups sliced, chunked or quartered turnips

1 lb | 450 g baby portobello mushrooms, cleaned, stemmed and quartered
Fresh, chopped Italian parsley
4 tablespoon | 55 g salted butter
1 tablespoon | 20 ml olive oil, for the Dutch oven

Method:

1. Preheat the oven to 350 °F/175 °C.
2. Coat a Dutch oven with olive oil and bring to medium-high heat.
3. Sprinkle the chuck roast liberally with salt, add it to the Dutch oven and brown it on all sides. Remove from the pan and reserve.
4. Lower the heat to medium and add the celery, onions and crushed red pepper to the pan. Sprinkle the vegetables with salt and cook until they are soft and begin to caramelize on the edges, about 8 to 10 minutes.
5. Add garlic and cook for 1 to 2 minutes. Remove the cooked veggies from the pot and reserve.
6. Place seared roast back in the Dutch oven, cover with reserved veggies. Pour in the wine and enough of the chicken stock to almost cover the meat. Taste and adjust the seasoning if needed. Toss in the bay leaves and thyme bundle. Cover the pan and bake for 1 hour.
7. Remove the pan from the oven, turn the meat over and add more stock if needed.
8. Continue to check on the meat hourly for doneness and to add more liquid if necessary.
9. When meat is nearly fall-apart tender, remove the pan from the oven and gently lift the meat from the pan to a plate.
10. Add the turnips to the liquid, and add any additional stock you still have reserved. Taste and adjust seasonings.
11. Place the meat on top of the liquid and veggies. Return to oven and continue to bake until turnips are fork tender.
12. Remove the pan from the oven. Add the mushrooms to the pan. Return to oven and bake an additional 15 minutes or until the mushrooms are soft.
13. Add a few pats of butter to the top of the meat and sprinkle with fresh, chopped

parsley. Serve directly from the roasting pan. No need for fancy plating for this homey meal.

Variation: Omit the turnips and spoon the meat and other veggies with the pan juice in a bowl over a serving of Mende's Cauliflower Mash.

* Check the chicken stock doesn't contain nightshades (spices, chilli, cayenne) or gluten and has very little carbohydrates.

Gluten free option | Egg free | Nut free | Nightshade free option

Serving size	Protein	Fat	Total Carbs	Net Carbs
9 oz 257 g	32.8 g	35.8 g	4.9 g	3.3 g

WE WISH YOU

Healthiest of Holidays

AND

HAPPY NEW YEAR

Ham Oven Baked

Mende

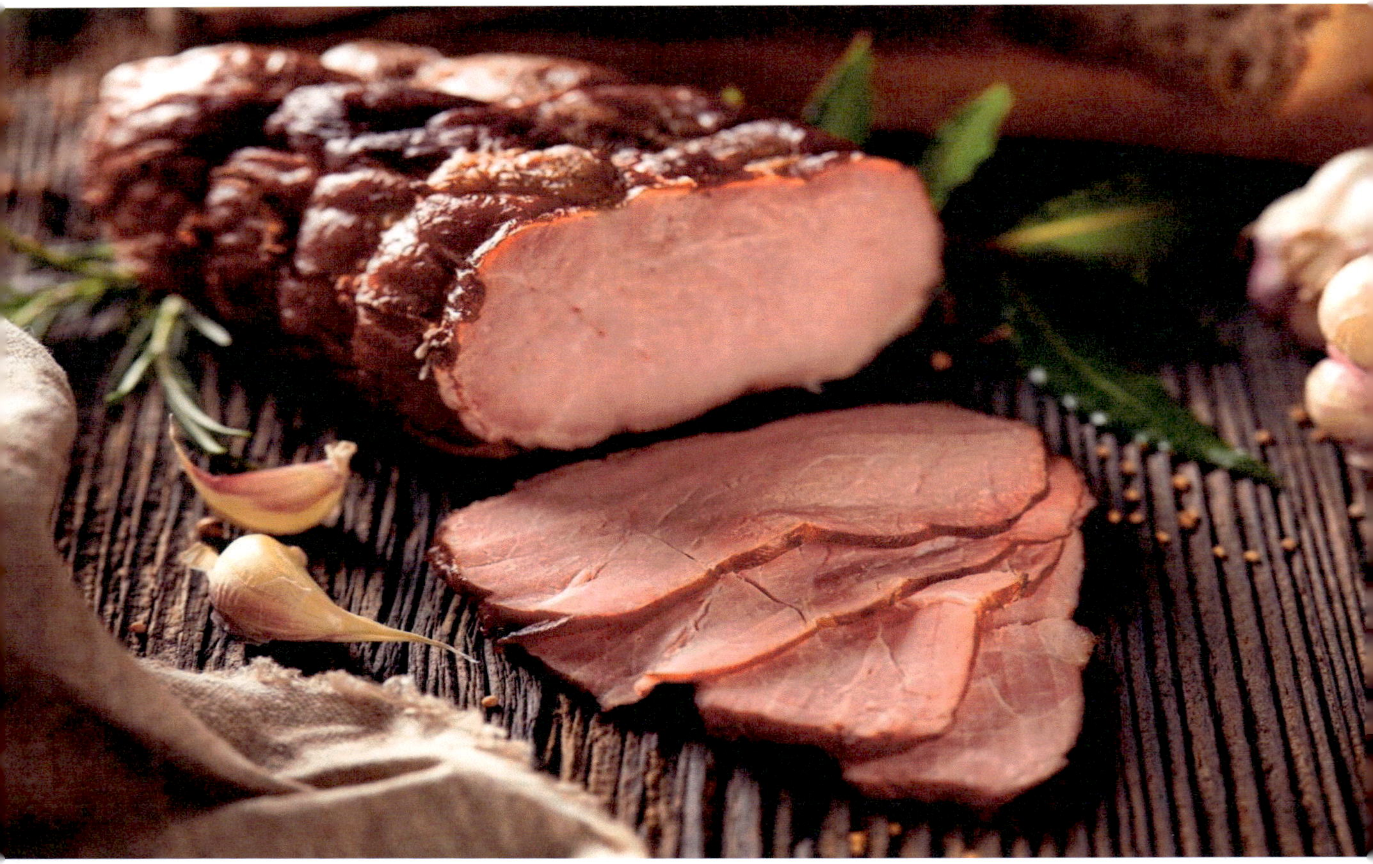

Servings: 10

Ingredients:

35 oz | 1kg fully-cooked smoked ham
½ cup extra virgin olive oil mayonnaise or avocado oil mayonnaise (Primal Kitchens brand is widely available)
1 cup dijon or stone-ground mustard
2 tablespoons lemon juice 3-4 cloves of garlic, minced
½ teaspoon salt, or to taste
½ teaspoon pepper, or to taste

Method:

1. Read package directions for heating ham. Set oven to recommended temperature. Place ham in roaster pan.
2. In a mixing bowl, combine mayo, mustard, lemon juice, garlic, salt and pepper.
3. Brush or spread half of the mustard sauce over the surface of the ham.
4. Reserve the other half of the sauce for serving.
5. Bake for the recommended time.
6. Serve ham with additional mustard sauce.

*Check ham & mustard label for gluten free and nightshade free

Gluten free option | Nut free | Dairy free

Serving size	Protein	Fat	Total Carbs	Net Carbs
5 oz 143 g	19.2 g	11.7 g	4.4 g	3.6 g

Mushroom Cauliflower Risotto with Seared Shrimp

Courtesy of John Starchman, Chef of the Red Onion Cafe, Joplin, MO

Mende

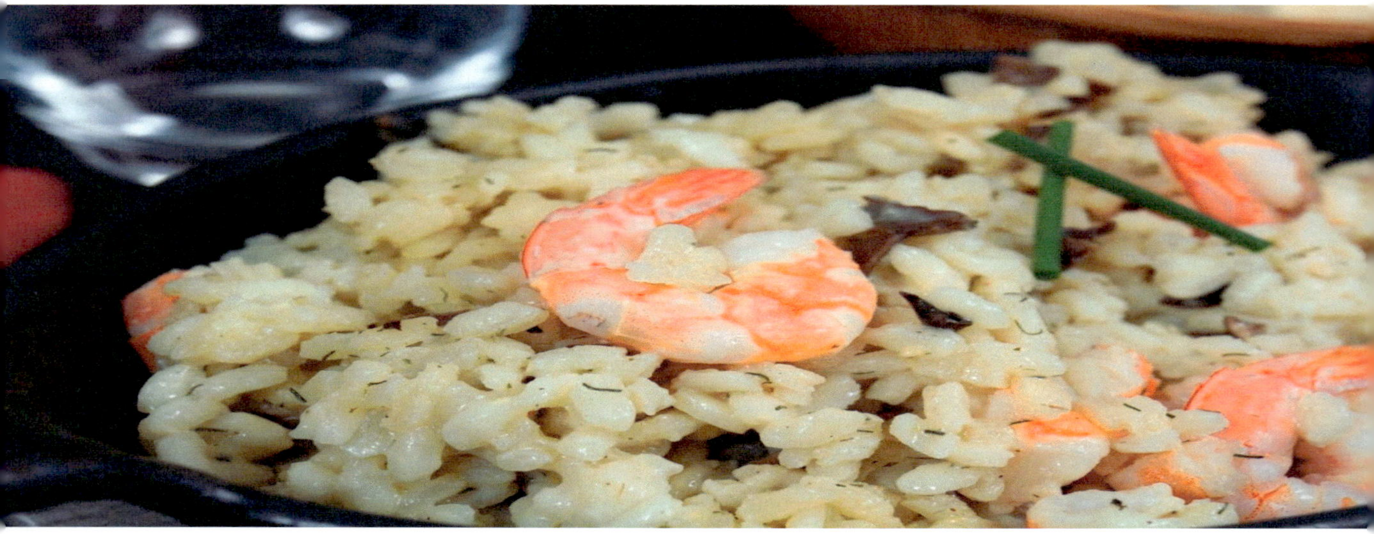

Servings: 4

Ingredients:

3 green onions, chopped
1 small bundle of fresh or dried oregano*, chopped finely
3 cloves bulb garlic, chopped finely
3 slices of thick-sliced bacon* (omit if vegetarian)
8 oz. | 225 g sliced baby portobello mushrooms
1 pound | 450 g jumbo raw peeled and deveined shrimp with tails on
1 pound | 450 g fresh cauliflower pearls or riced cauliflower
¾ cup heavy whipping cream**
½ cup sour cream**
½ cup | 50 g grated smoked gouda cheese
2 tablespoon salted butter

½ teaspoon garlic powder*
1 teaspoon smoked sea salt (or any salt), or to taste

¼ teaspoon cayenne pepper (substitute black pepper if nightshade intolerant), or to taste

Method:

1. In a medium sized frying pan saute mushrooms in butter and set them aside.
2. In the same frying pan, fry the bacon, remove from the pan, but reserve bacon grease.
3. Sear the shrimp in the bacon grease, 5-6 at a time, and set them aside, too.
4. Add cauliflower pearls to the hot bacon grease, then add chopped garlic, onion and fresh oregano along with some powdered garlic, cayenne or black pepper, and smoked sea salt (any salt will do, but this is extra special!)
5. When the cauliflower is nicely seared, add bacon and mushrooms. Pour in some heavy whipping cream and reduce, then give it a dollop of sour cream for good measure.
6. Continue to cook and stir until the creams are reduced and thickened, remove from heat, and sprinkle with grated smoked gouda cheese. Stir until the cheese begins to melt.
7. Place the risotto onto a plate and top with the cooked shrimp.

*If celiac ensure bacon not cross-contaminated with gluten. Check herb allergen list for gluten.
** Check for emulsifiers and check allergen list for gluten.

Gluten free option | Egg free | Nut free |
Nightshade free option | Pescatarian (omit bacon)

Serving size	Protein	Fat	Total Carbs	Net Carbs
12.8 oz 363 g	37.6 g	26.3 g	11.1 g	7.7 g

Salmon with Cripsy Skin, Hollandaise Sauce and Toasted Almonds

Megan

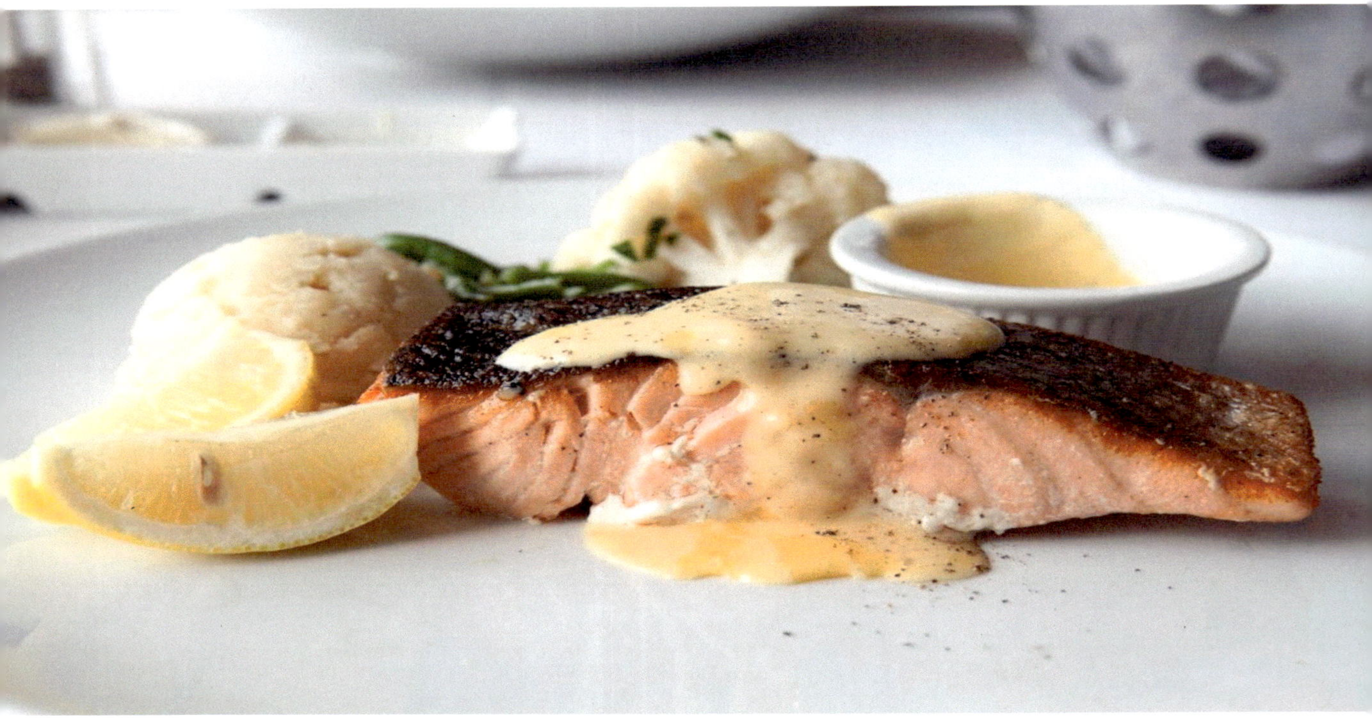

Servings: 4

Ingredients:

4 wild Atlantic salmon fillets, medium size (no more than 150 g) & skin on
2 oz | 60 g flaked almonds (omit for nut free)
1 stick | 114 g salted butter, for hollandaise sauce
1 tablespoon salted butter, for toasting the nuts
2 oz | 56 g cream cheese*, room temperature

3 egg yolks, medium size, room temperature
2 tablespoon lemon juice
¼ teaspoon of salt, or to taste
1 tablespoon fresh chives, finely chopped or cut with scissors
30 ml extra virgin olive oil, for pan frying the fish

Method:

1. Remove fish from the fridge 20 minutes prior to cooking to get to room temperature. Keep covered in a sealed container.
2. On the stovetop, place the butter in a small sized frying pan on medium heat, and once melted and bubbling add the flaked almonds.
3. Turn the temperature down to low and stir the almonds once you can see them start to brown. Keep stirring until a light golden brown all over. Set aside on a plate lined with paper towels .
4. Place the cream cheese and egg yolks into a tall container or food processor. Whisk together until combined.
5. In a container or jug with a spout, melt the butter in the microwave or on the stovetop until just melted, remove and add/combine the lemon juice and salt.
6. Gradually whisk (or blend with a stick blender or food processor) the butter into the cream cheese and egg yolk mixture, stopping intermittently until the butter is fully combined. Cover container or jug with a lid or foil to keep warm.
7. Pat fish all over with paper towel until dry, and lightly salt the fish on both sides.
8. Heat a large sized frying pan on high heat for a minute or two, add olive oil then add the salmon, skin side down (the pan should sizzle when the fish is added).
9. Turn the heat down to medium and cook for approx. 4 minutes or until the skin looks a golden brown, then turn the fish over.
10. Cook for a further 4 minutes or until a lovely golden colour, then flip back to the skin side.
11. Turn the heat down to low, cover the frying pan with a lid and cook for a further 3 to 5 minutes to allow the fish to cook through. It is ready when you

see the colour turns from a dark to a soft pink in thickest part of the fish. Remove immediately from the pan - fish will dry out if you overcook it.

12. Plate the fish and add 2 to 3 tablespoons of hollandaise over the top. Garnish with toasted almonds and chopped chives.

* Check the brand doesn't contain emulsifiers.

Gluten free | Egg free | Nut free option | Nightshade free | Pescatarian

Serving size	Protein	Fat	Total Carbs	Net Carbs
6.6 oz 189 g	29.1 g	43.5 g	6 g	4.5 g

Fat gives things flavor.

~Julia Child

Simple Spinach Pie

Raeann

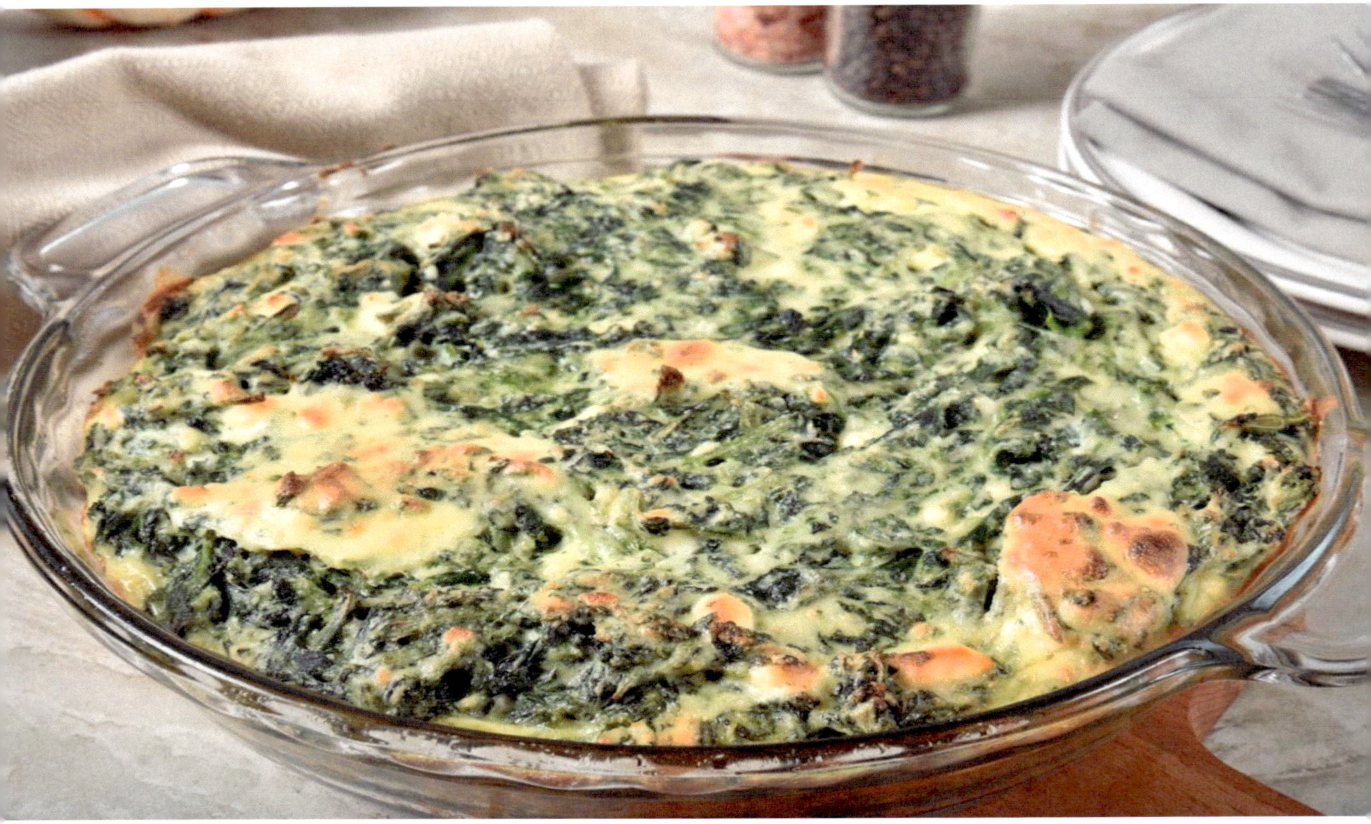

Servings: 8

Ingredients:

1 bunch spinach, washed and drained
5 eggs, beaten
2 ½ cups of cheese, grated* (Swiss, Asiago, Manchego, Parmesan or any cheese, or cheese combo, you like) *Grate the cheese yourself to avoid starchy additives in pre grated cheese or read labels carefully.*

½ teaspoon onion powder*
¼ teaspoon garlic powder*
3 dashes | 3 g natural salt, or to taste
2 dashes | 2 g pepper, or to taste

Method:

1. Preheat oven to 375°F/190°C.
2. Combine ingredients and pile into a greased 9 inch pie plate.
3. Bake for 30 minutes or until edges are golden brown.

*Check herbs and packaged grated cheese allergen list for gluten. Check packaged grated cheese for potato starch for nightshade intolerance and extra carbs.

Gluten free | Nut free | Nightshade free | Vegetarian

Serving size	Protein	Fat	Total Carbs	Net Carbs
4.1 oz/117g	16.2 g	12.2 g	3.6 g	3.5 g

Tourtiere - Christmas Eve Pie

Raeann

Tourtiere is a French-Canadian holiday meat pie traditionally served on Christmas Eve.

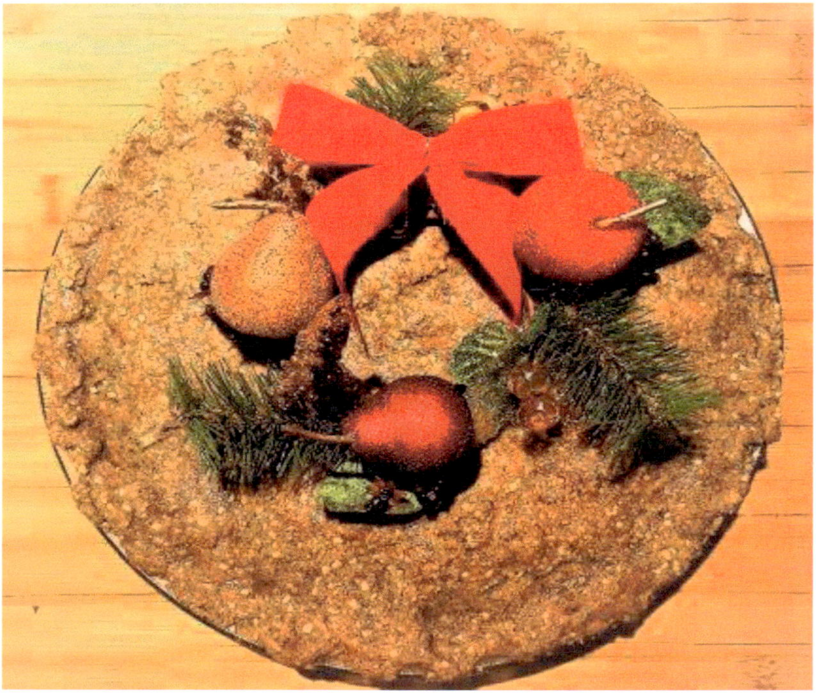

photo courtesy of Raeann Sparks

Servings: 8

Ingredients:

For the Low Carb Bake Mix:

4 cups almond meal (or almond flour)
4 cups raw sunflower seeds, ground
1 cup flax seeds, ground (or flax meal)
1 cup chia seeds, ground
½ cup coconut flour, ground
1 cup hemp hearts, ground
¼ cup psyllium husks, ground
4 teaspoon of baking soda

NOTE: A chemical reaction between the baking soda and the raw sunflower seeds can create a green colour with time. Omit the baking soda to prevent this if desired.

For the Pastry:

4 cups Low Carb Bake Mix
½ teaspoon natural salt
½ teaspoon baking powder (gluten and aluminium free)
½ cup lard, tallow or butter
2 large eggs
1 teaspoon Apple Cider Vinegar

For the Filling:

3 lbs | 1.35 kg ground pork
1 lb | 450 g ground turkey *
½ lb | 225 g pork or turkey organs such as liver, kidney, gizzard, and/or heart **
1 chorizo sausage, casing removed (omit if nightshade intolerant)
⅓ cup onion, roughly chopped
3 cloves garlic, peeled
1 cup water
1 teaspoon natural salt
1 tablespoon ground sage
½ teaspoon ground thyme
1 teaspoon celery seed
2 teaspoon ground allspice
2 teaspoon ground cinnamon
½ teaspoon ground nutmeg
½ teaspoon ground cloves
½ teaspoon ground ginger
(source certified gluten free spices where required)
2 cups cooked cauliflower, puréed
3 tablespoon bacon grease (or salted butter, duck or chicken fat)

Method for Low Carb Bake Mix:

1. Grind seeds in a food processor or coffee grinder.
2. Mix all ingredients together in a bowl.
3. Keep in an air-tight container in the freezer and use as needed.

Method for Pastry:

1. Mix the dry ingredients very well.
2. Cut the cold lard into pea size cubes and place individually in the dry ingredients.

3. Cut the fat into the mixture with a pastry cutter or fork until it resembles rice with some larger bits of fat
4. Whisk eggs and ACV together in a separate bowl and mix into pastry until it forms a dough.
5. Add small amounts of ice water if the dough needs more moisture to stick together.
6. Separate the dough into four disks for bottom and top of pies, making the bottom disks a little bigger.
7. Chill in the refrigerator while making the filling.

Method for Filling:

1. Soak organ meat in Apple Cider Vinegar.
2. Add all other meats to a thick bottom pot. Use your hands to mix them well making sure there are no clumps.
3. Trim membranes from the organ meat, discard the trimmings and chop the meat into chunks small enough for the food processor.
4. Grind the organ meats, onion and garlic together using a food processor. Add the mixture to the other meat in the pot and mix well.
5. Add water to the pot, bring to a slow boil, turn the heat down and simmer.
6. Stir in salt, herbs and spices. Frequent stirring will stop it from browning or clumping. Simmer for 30 minutes, or until it is well cooked and the water is incorporated.
7. Mix cauliflower purée and bacon grease in and set to cool while rolling out the pastry for two 9″ pies.

Method for Assembling:

1. Preheat oven to 350 °F/175 °C.
2. Roll bottom crust between two pieces of wax paper flipping once or twice.
3. Peel off one wax paper and flip into a 9 inch pie plate.
4. Peel the other wax paper away, repair tears and trim edges.
5. Fill the bottom pie crust.

6. Roll the top crust and peel and flip onto the top of the pie.
7. Crimp Edges. Wash with beaten egg if desired.
8. Make the second pie. Freeze one for later use if desired.
9. Cover the edges of the pie with foil to prevent burning the crust edges.
10. Bake for 50 minutes or until the crust is golden brown. Serve warm.

TIP: Thaw the frozen pie overnight in the refrigerator or for two hours prior to baking.

** You can use turkey leftovers removed from the carcass before making bone broth and ground in your food processor. Or even better, pick the bones and hard plant materials out of the strainings from your Thanksgiving turkey bone broth. Squeeze and drain well. Freeze in 1 lb bags to use later in your Christmas Tourtiere. Thaw and grind in your food processor with your onion, garlic and offal. (See Turkey Bone Broth recipe)*

*** This is a great way to start adding the planet's most nutrient dense and nutrient accessible food to your diet. Begin with heart, because when ground well, it adds texture and can't be detected flavour wise. Kidney and liver have more flavour, but soaking in the ACV helps mellow the flavour, which I find delicious. Ground liver is the best meat glue going. It really helps your pie filling hold it's shape. Growing up, my family always used our traditional northern English turkey stuffing recipe which called for grinding the giblets into the recipe. Giblets and spices smell like Christmas to me.*

*Check ingredient allergen labels for gluten free.

Gluten free option | Dairy free | Nightshade free option

Serving size	Protein	Fat	Total Carbs	Net Carbs
8.5 oz 240 g	30.6 g	46.3 g	11.9 g	4.9 g

Turkey Roasted

Mende

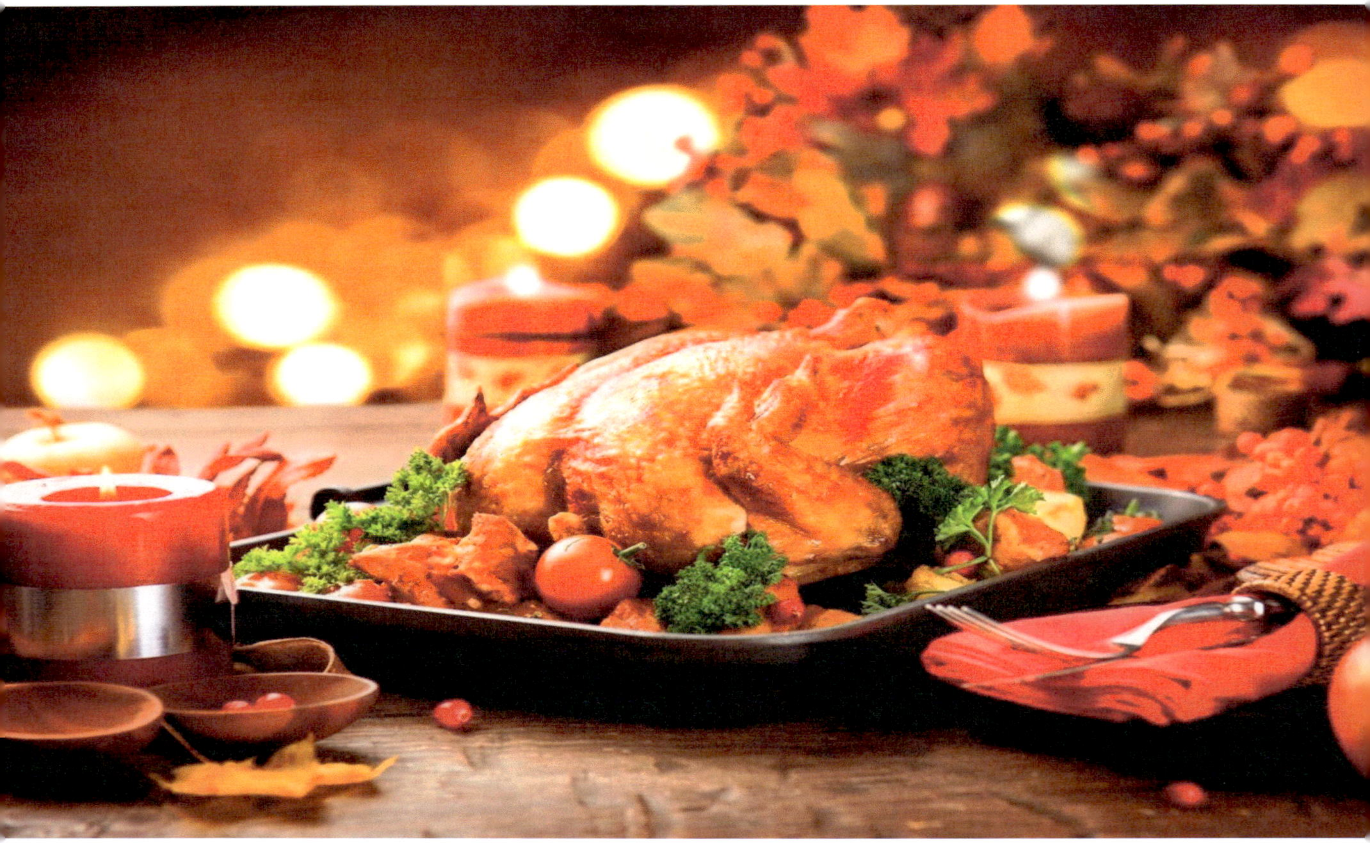

Servings: 15, depending on the size of the turkey

Ingredients:

1 x 12 lb l 5.5 kg turkey - *match size of turkey to the size of your crowd. I figure 1 ½ pounds of turkey weight (including bone weight) per person, and allows for left-overs if less than 15 people.*

Ingredients for Brine:

This needs to be prepared at least 12 hours before you plan to START cooking the turkey! Be prepared to double the brine recipe depending on the size of your turkey and the brining container.

A container large enough to hold the turkey plus the brine. The turkey must be completely submerged in the brine. I use a small ice chest.

1 cup Kosher salt
½ gallon hot water
Enough ice + cold water to add to hot water to make 2 gallons iced brine
1 head of garlic, crushed (no need to peel)
1 tablespoon whole black peppercorns
1 teaspoon ground allspice
1 bunch fresh rosemary, bruised (or 1 tablespoon dried rosemary)
1 bunch fresh sage, bruised (or 1 tablespoon dried, rubbed sage)
1 bundle of fresh thyme (or 1 tablespoon dried thyme)
2 or 3 bay leaves, fresh or dried

Note: Check spice allergen lists for gluten.

Ingredients for the turkey cavity aromatics:

Celery leaves and spindly stems from the top of a bunch of celery - *I save these when I prepare the celery for the dressing recipe.*

1 medium onion, quartered
3 or 4 cloves of garlic, smashed
1 small carrot, cut into chunks
1 bunch each: fresh rosemary, sage, and thyme

Ingredients for the butter rub for the outside of the turkey:

½ stick (4 tablespoon or 55 g) salted butter, softened (for dairy-free substitute ¼ cup olive oil)
1 teaspoon poultry seasoning
½ teaspoon ground sweet or smoked paprika (omit if nightshade intolerant)

Note: check spices for gluten

Method for the Brine:

1. Prepare brine at least 12 hours before you plan to START cooking the turkey.
2. In a large saucepan or stock pot, combine hot water and salt.
3. Cook and stir over medium-high heat until all the salt is dissolved. Set aside to cool.
4. Add garlic, peppercorns, allspice, rosemary, sage, thyme and bay leaves to hot brine.
5. Open turkey packaging, remove neck and giblets. Reserve these for making broth.
6. Wash the inside of the turkey cavity, if necessary. Let the turkey drain in/over the sink while you finish the brine. Wash hands.
7. Pour the cooled brine (it will still be warm but no longer boiling hot) into your large container, add the ice to make 2 gallons of ice and brine.
8. Gently place the turkey, breast side down, into the brine. If the turkey isn't floating in the brine, you may need to mix up more iced brine water (no need to add more herbs and spices). This will depend greatly upon the size of the container and the size of the turkey. I prefer to use an ice chest for this since I usually don't have the refrigerator space for the brining container. The iced salt water keeps the turkey at a food-safe cold temperature.
9. Brine for 12-14 hours (overnight).

Method for the turkey cavity aromatics:

1. Be sure to start turkey preparation to allow for appropriate roasting time.
2. Most grocery-store turkeys have a roasting time guide based on weight. If yours does not, figure about 20 minutes per pound roasting time.
3. Preheat oven to 325 degrees Fahrenheit.
4. Remove turkey from the brine and rinse to remove bits of spices and herbs.
5. Place turkey on the rack of a large roaster pan.
6. Stuff the inside cavity with aromatics. You may need to cut the vegetables into smaller pieces to make them fit, but don't worry about making them pretty. Fit

as many of the dried herbs and aromatic vegetables as possible inside the turkey.

7. Dry the turkey skin with paper towels.

Method for the butter rub for the outside of the turkey:

1. Mix poultry seasoning and paprika (omit paprika if nightshade intolerant) with softened butter to make a paste.
2. Rub paste over the turkey skin, or slide your hand under the skin and spread the paste directly on the breast meat under the skin.
3. Place the giblets with a cup of water or broth in the bottom of the roaster pan.

Method for roasting the turkey:

1. Roast recommended amount of time based on weight.
2. You may find it necessary to make a tent of aluminum foil to protect the wing tips during the first few hours of cooking.
3. When done, let the turkey rest at least 20 minutes.
4. Transfer the bird to a serving platter before carving.
5. The aromatics in the bird cavity are not meant to be eaten, but they, along with the turkey carcass and roasted giblets, make excellent turkey stock, so don't throw them away.

The drippings from the bottom of the roasting pan will be both broth and fat. Refrigerate them to remove the fat easily from the broth. The fat may be reserved for later cooking (great for roasting vegetables), and the gelatinous broth can be heated and combined with heavy cream, sour cream or creme fraiche to make a delicious drizzling sauce for the turkey meat. There should be little to no waste when roasting a turkey!

Macro note: You need to add turkey stuffing onto the macro count, if using.

Gluten free option | Egg free | Nut free |
Dairy free option | Nightshade free option

Serving size	Protein	Fat	Total Carbs	Net Carbs
4.4 oz. 124 g	26 g	9.9 g	0.3 g	0.3 g

Happy
THANKSGIVING

Turkey Dressing with Chestnuts

Catherine

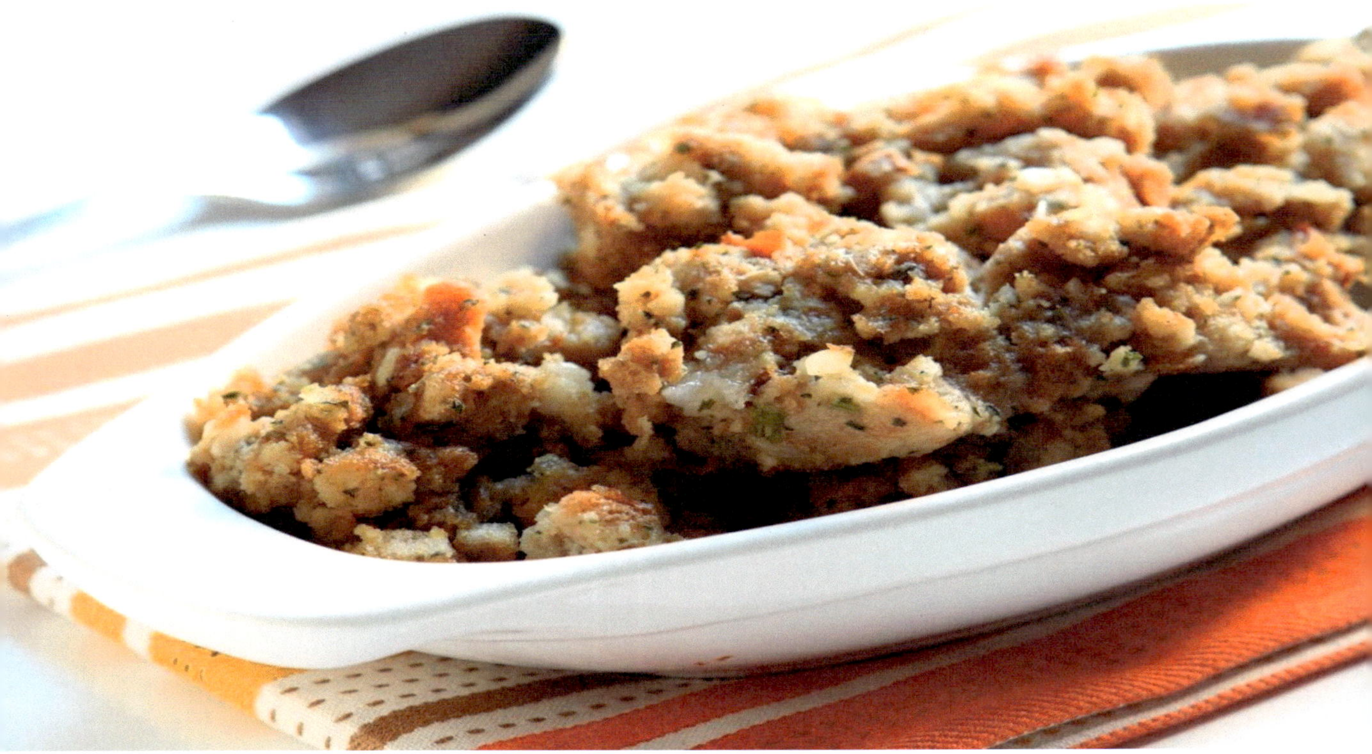

Servings: 20

Ingredients:

10 oz | 285 g package of bacon*
2-3 lbs | 720 g sausage - I use Italian hot sausages for the spice, use just the meat remove the casings
2 packages, Pre-cooked Italian chestnuts (each package is 3.5 oz | 100 g)*
4 oz | 114 g salted butter added to bacon and sausage drippings
1 bunch of celery, diced
2 onions, large sized, diced
6 carrots, large sized, diced
5 cups cauliflower rice
½ teaspoon salt, or to taste
½ teaspoon coarse black pepper
2 tablespoon sage

Method:

1. In a large frying pan sauté the bacon until crispy then cut into small pieces.
2. Add in the sausage meat (remove casings if needed) on medium heat until cooked.
3. Add in the butter, celery, onion, carrots, cauliflower rice, sage, salt and pepper and sauté.
4. Cook and stir to evenly distribute.
5. Dice 2 packages of pre-cooked Italian chestnuts into small pieces. Add the diced chestnuts and cook another 5-7 minutes.
6. Then you are ready to stuff the bird and/or roast in a separate baking dish - I usually add in another sprinkle of sage or turkey spices on top with a few dots of butter.
7. Roast in the bird or alongside the bird until done - 30-40 minutes in a medium oven -300° F/150° C.

*Check bacon, sausage and sage for gluten, and for spices/cayenne/chili for nightshade intolerance

Gluten free option | Dairy free | Nightshade free option

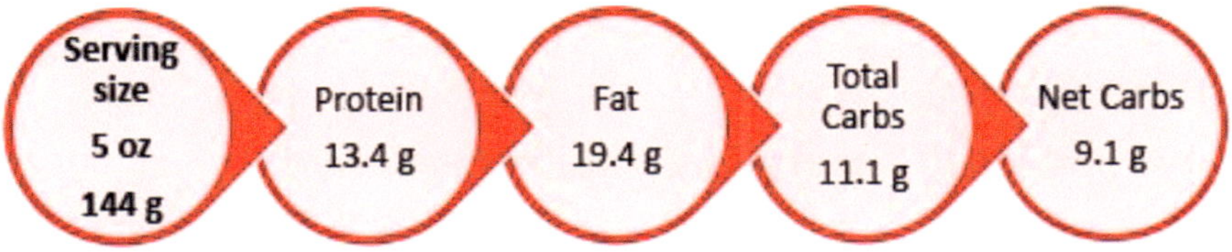

Turkey Dressing with Cheesy Skillet Bread

Mende

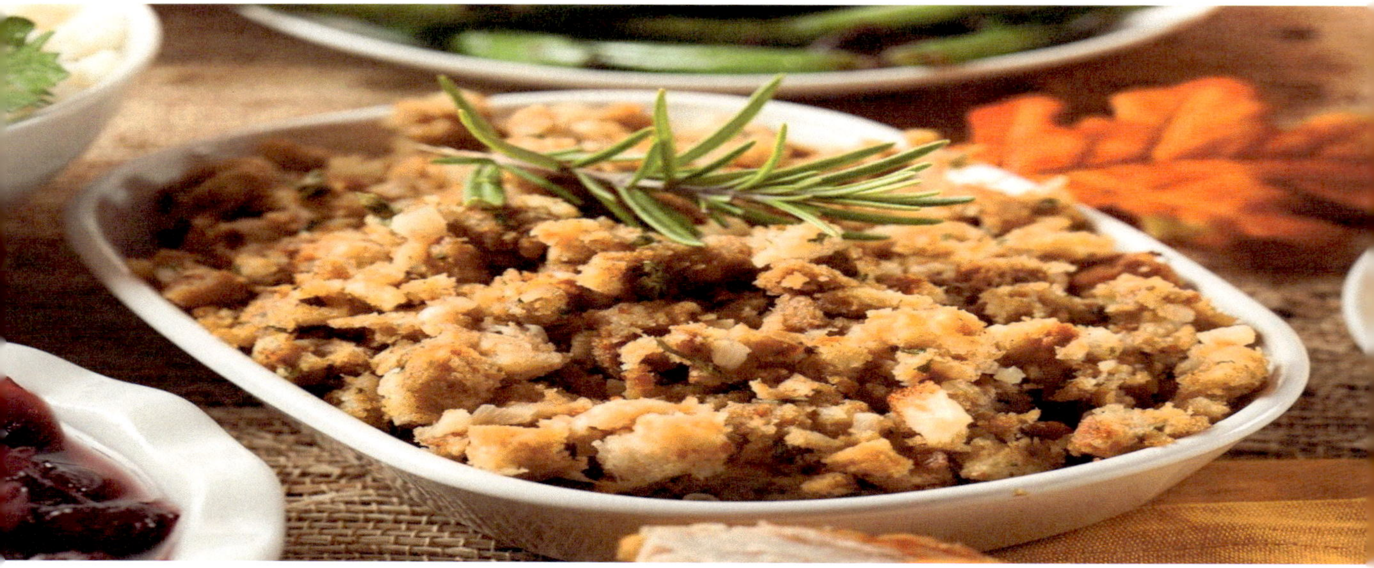

Servings: 12

Ingredients:

1 batch Cheesy Skillet Bread (made at least 1 day in advance)
1 stick | 114 g butter, plus more for baking dish
1 ½ cups chopped celery (save trimmings for turkey preparation)
½ medium onion, chopped
½ cup chicken or vegetable broth*, or reserved turkey drippings (fat removed)
¼ cup chopped Italian parsley (or 2 tablespoon dried*)
1 tablespoon chopped fresh sage (or 1 teaspoon dried*)
1 tablespoon chopped fresh rosemary (or 1 teaspoon dried*)
1 tablespoon chopped fresh thyme (or 1 teaspoon dried*)
¼ teaspoon black pepper
½ teaspoon salt, or to taste

Optional ingredient: 1 pound | 450 g cooked and drained sage breakfast sausage (check for gluten & spices if nightshade intolerant).

Method:

1. Cut bread into ½-inch cubes and spread onto a parchment paper-lined baking sheet.
2. Bake at 300 degrees for about 20 minutes, turning as needed, until dry.
3. While bread is drying, in a large skillet, saute celery and onion with salt in butter until soft.
4. Stir in parsley, sage, rosemary, thyme and pepper. Remove from heat.
5. Place bread cubes into a large mixing bowl. Pour butter and veggies over the bread.
6. Add sausage, if using. Toss to combine.
7. Pour chicken broth or turkey drippings over the bread mixture. Stir. If bread still seems dry, add a bit more liquid.
8. Press into a buttered baking dish. Bake at 400 degrees until the top is lightly browned.

*Check herbs for gluten, check broth for gluten and spices if nightshade intolerant.

Gluten free option | Nightshade free option | Lacto/Ovo/Vegetarian option

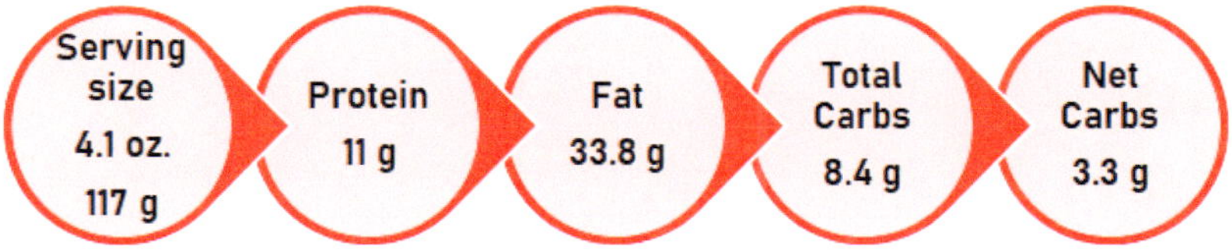

Turkey Bone Broth

Raeann

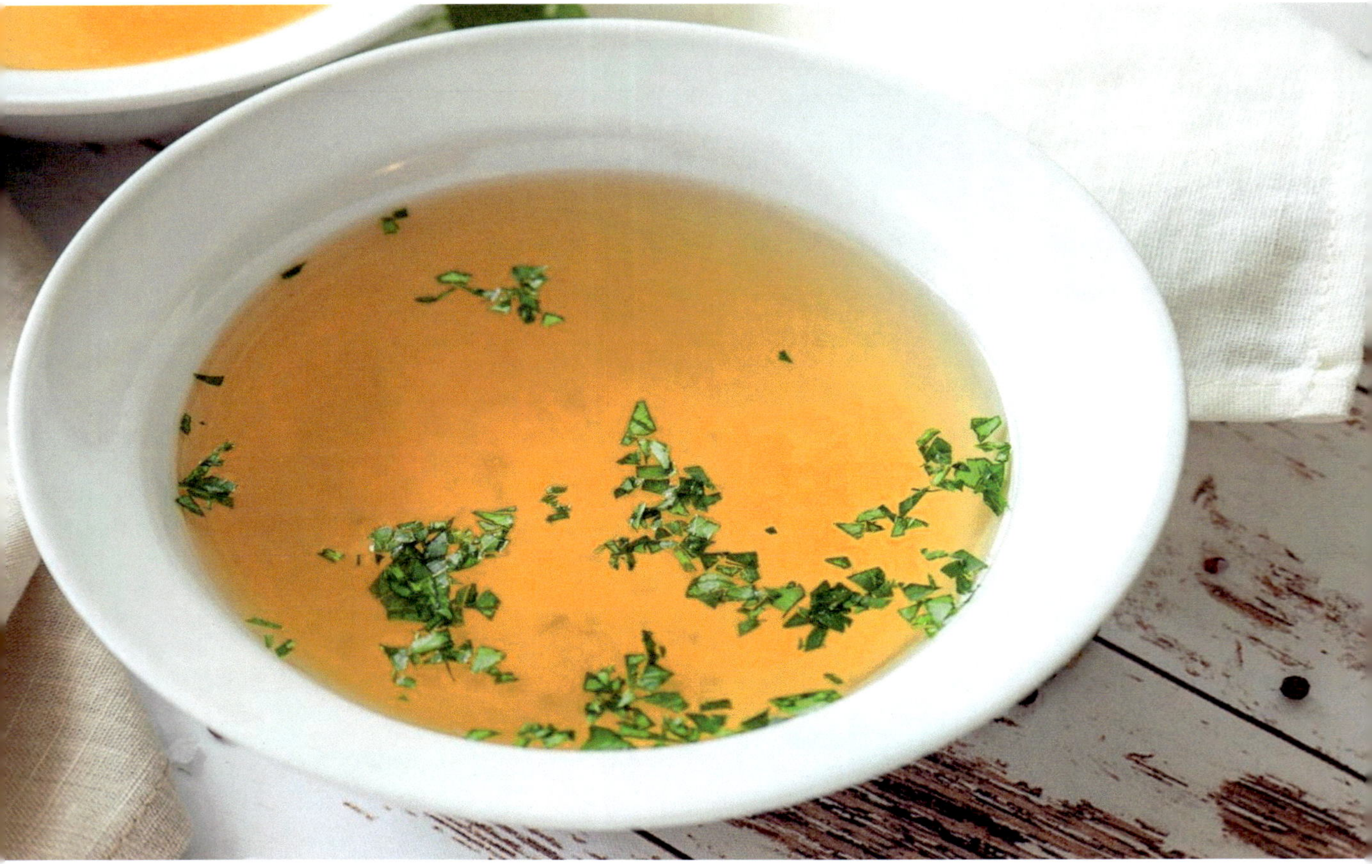

Servings: 40 cups

Ingredients:

1 x roasted turkey carcass 2 tablespoon natural salt
6 tablespoon apple cider vinegar (ACV)
Vegetable peelings, cores and stalks, well washed - *I use ones reserved from holiday dinner preparations*
1 tablespoon poultry seasoning (check allergen listing is gluten free)
10.5 litres water

Method:

1. In a large stock pot add the turkey carcass to the water, salt and ACV.
2. Bring to a boil, reduce heat to low and simmer for 24 hours or longer until the bones are softening.
3. Add the seasonings and vegetable scraps.
4. Simmer for another hour or more.
5. Taste and adjust the salt and seasonings, if required.
6. Cool, strain and freeze for use in soups, sauces, and as a fasting or fast-breaking drink.

Turkey Soup

Catherine

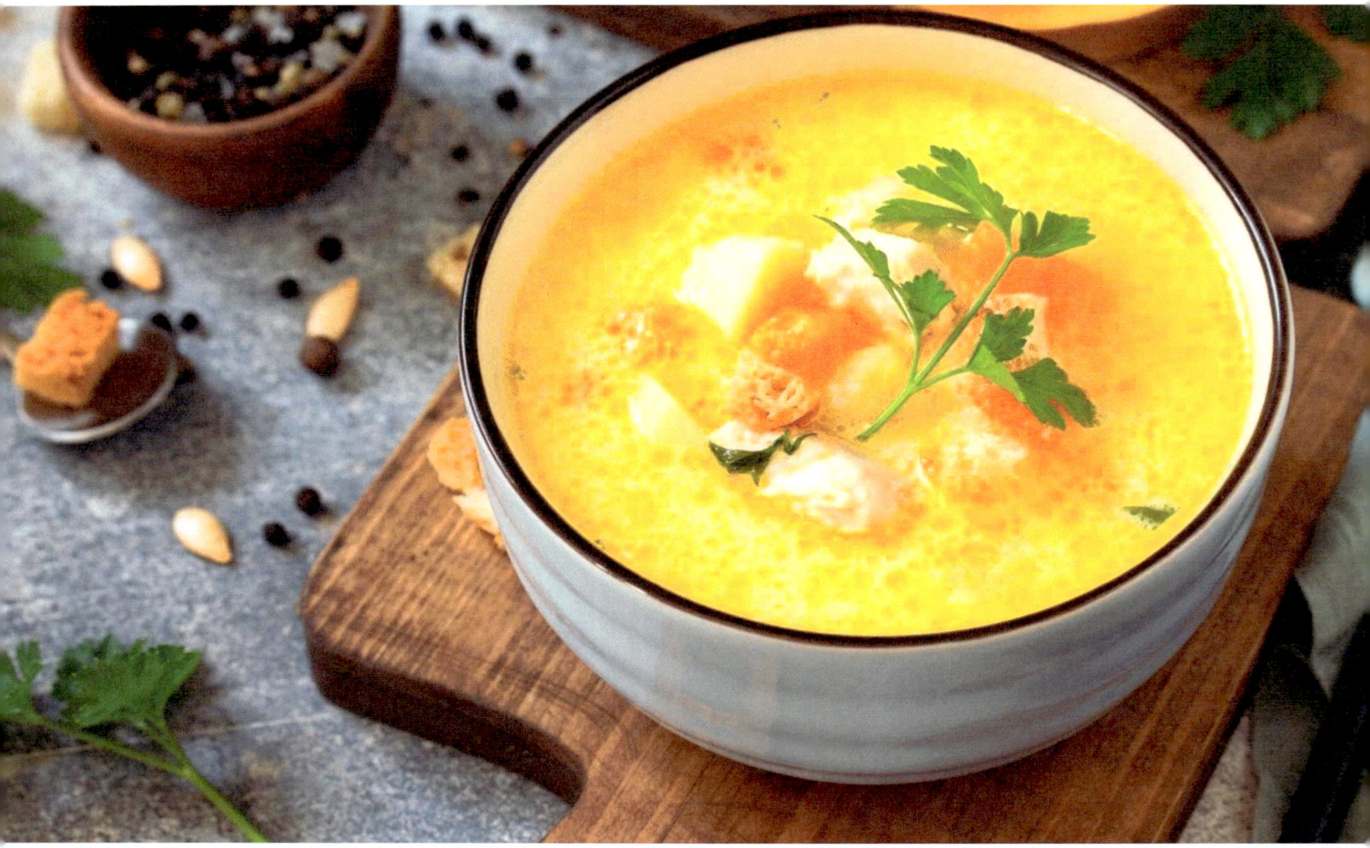

Servings: 6

Ingredients:

1 tablespoon extra virgin olive oil
2 tablespoon butter - *I like Kerrygold from grass-fed cow's milk butter*
1 large onion, minced
4 celery stalks, chopped
3 large carrots, chopped
6 cups turkey bone broth (see recipe)
1 cup turkey meat (reserved from cooking bone broth)
2 tablespoon natural salt, to taste
Parsley, to serve

Variation: Add 2 cups greens, kale, spinach, escarole, mushrooms, to taste (not included in macro count).

Method:

1. Heat the olive oil and butter in a large pot over medium-high heat.
2. Add the onion and cook for 5 minutes.
3. Add the carrot and cook until it begins to brown, about 5 minutes.
4. Add the celery, turkey bone broth, and the reserved turkey meat and bring to a boil.
5. Simmer for 10-15 minutes, or until the carrots and celery are soft.
6. Season to taste generously with salt.

Gluten free | Egg free | Nut free | Nightshade free

Serving size	Protein	Fat	Total Carbs	Net Carbs
4.1 oz 117 g	11.9 g	7 g	8.6 g	6.8 g

You don't have to cook fancy
or complicated masterpieces -
just good food
from fresh ingredients.

~Julia Child

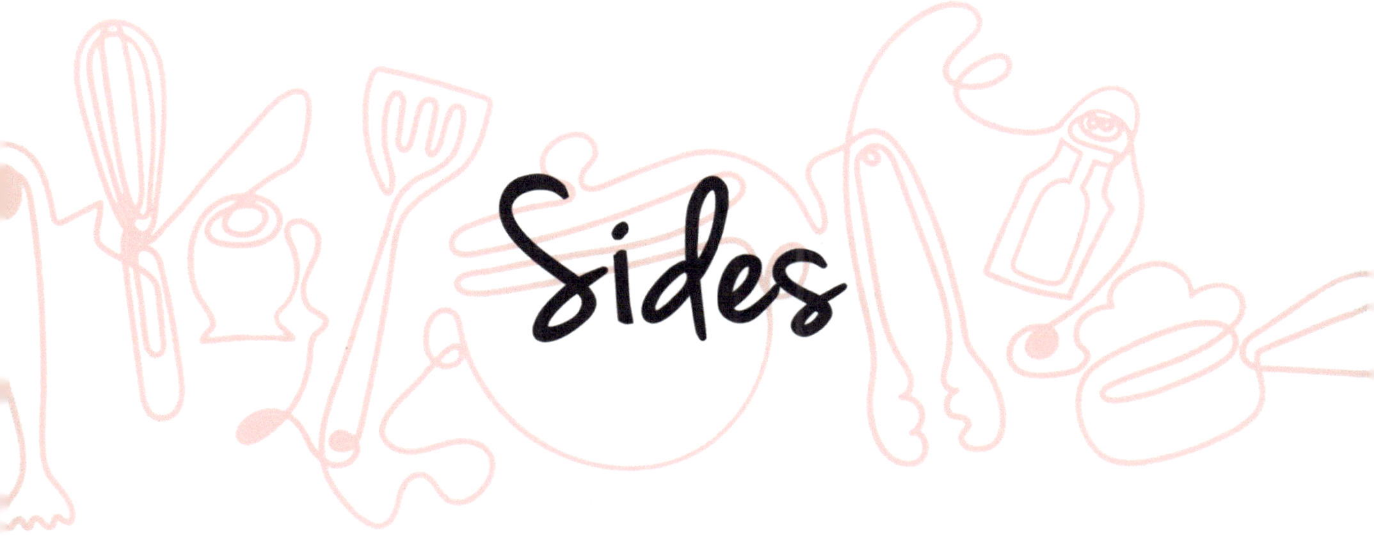

Sides

"When a radish can be a radish, you can be you! And when the radish is good enough being a radish, then you are good enough just being you."

~Edward Espe Brown

Asparagus and Mushrooms

Courtesy John Starchman, Red Onion Cafe, Joplin, Missouri

Mende

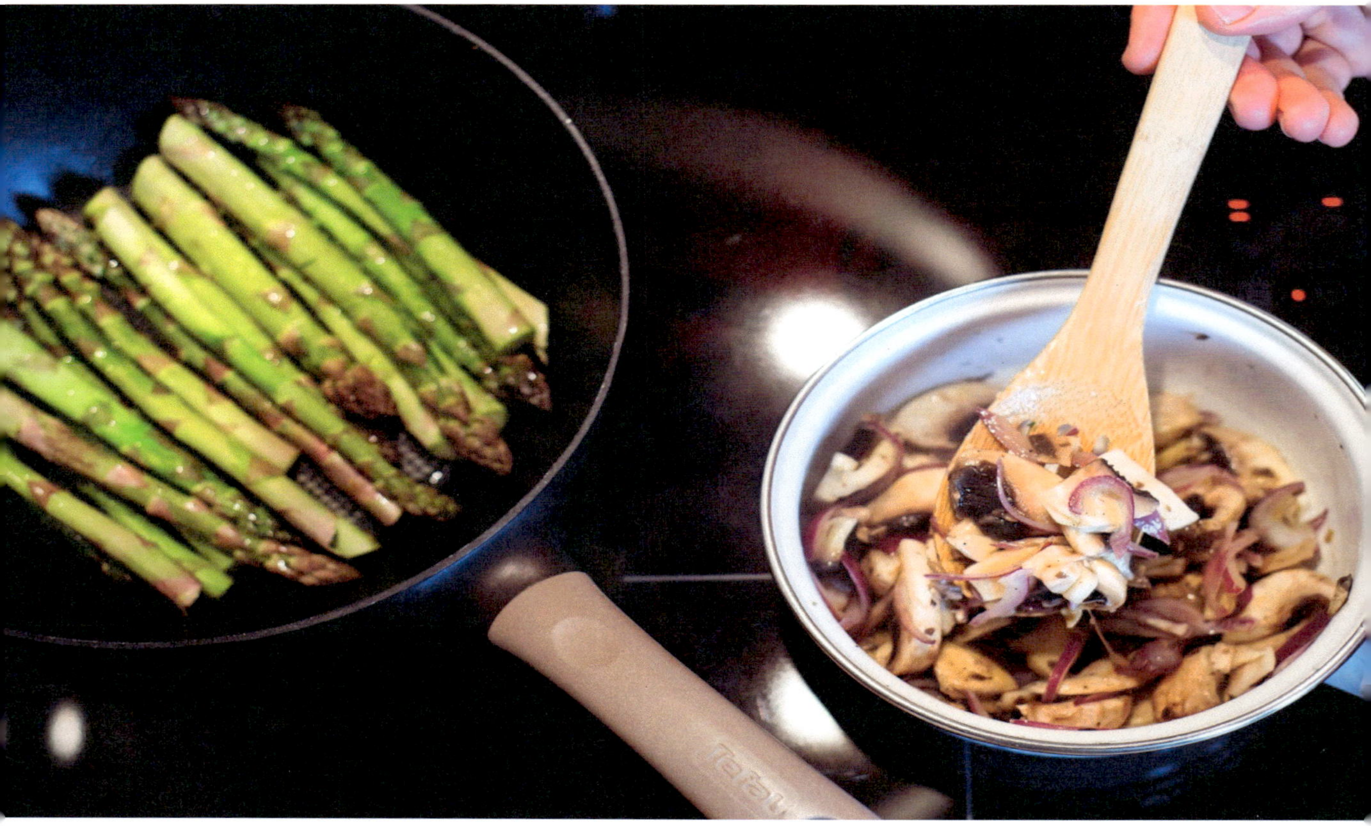

Servings: 8

Ingredients:

1 pound | 450 g asparagus, cut into 1 inch pieces and discard any woody parts of stem
1 pound | 450 g sliced button or baby portobello mushrooms
1 tablespoon fresh thyme
½ cup heavy cream*
¼ teaspoon smoked paprika (omit for nightshade sensitivity)
½ teaspoon granulated garlic**
½ teaspoon salt (or to taste)
½ stick (4 tablespoons) salted butter
1 cup shredded cheese**, optional (my favorite is smoked gouda)
a dash (about ⅛ teaspoon) of Cayenne Pepper (may substitute black pepper for nightshade sensitivity)

Method:

1. In a large skillet, sauté mushrooms in butter and salt over medium-high heat.
2. Add the asparagus to the pan, sauté for 30 seconds.
3. When they turn bright green add the heavy cream, smoked paprika, if using, and garlic.
4. Add heavy cream and cook to reduce until thickened.
5. Add a dash of cayenne pepper (or black pepper), and fresh thyme, give it a stir.
6. Remove from heat. Stir in ½ cup cheese, if using.
7. Top with remaining ½ cup of cheese and broil for a few minutes until the cheese is bubbly, if desired.

*Check cream for emulsifiers.
**Check allergen list for gluten.
***Check for potato starch if nightshade intolerant and to avoid additional carbs.

Gluten free option | Egg free | Nut free | Nightshade free option | Lacto Vegetarian

Serving size	Protein	Fat	Total Carbs	Net Carbs
5.3 oz 149 g	6.1 g	16 g	6.4 g	3.5 g

Brussel Sprouts Caramelized

Catherine

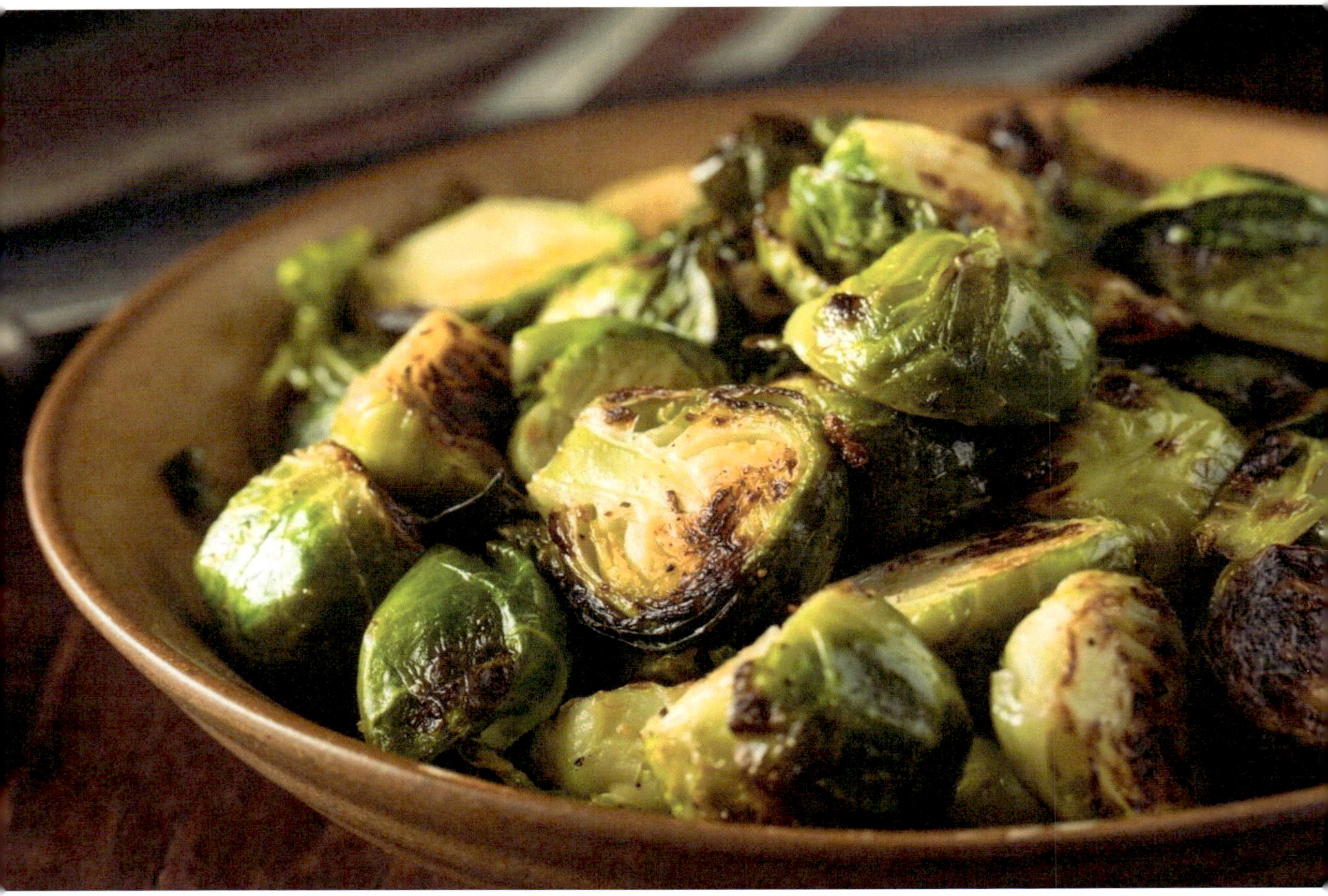

Servings: 8

Ingredients:

2 lbs | 900 g brussel sprouts (split in half)
4 slices of bacon*, chopped
1 teaspoon salt, to taste
1 teaspoon ground black pepper, to taste
1 stick | 114 g salted butter *(I like Kerrygold butter from grass-fed cow's milk)*

Method:

1. Preheat oven to 300 °F/150 °C.
2. Render the bacon in a large frying pan on medium heat.
3. Add the brussel sprouts in a roasting pan,
4. Add in salt, pepper, cut up pieces of butter.
5. Add in cut up bacon and bacon drippings.
6. Stir well.
7. Lower oven temperature to 250 °F/120 °C. Roast in a slow over for 1 ½ - 2 hours. The slow oven helps to caramelize the brussel sprouts.

Variation: Add ½ cup shredded cheese** the last 5-7 minutes in the oven and let melt. Onions and mushrooms are wonderful optional adds to this (not included in macro count).

*Check allergen warning for gluten free.
**Check for potato starch if nightshade intolerant

Gluten free option | Egg free | Nut free | Nightshade free

Serving size	Protein	Fat	Total Carbs	Net Carbs
4.6 oz 132 g	4.4 g	13.5 g	8.2 g	5.2 g

Cauliflower Mash (plain, loaded & casserole)

Mende

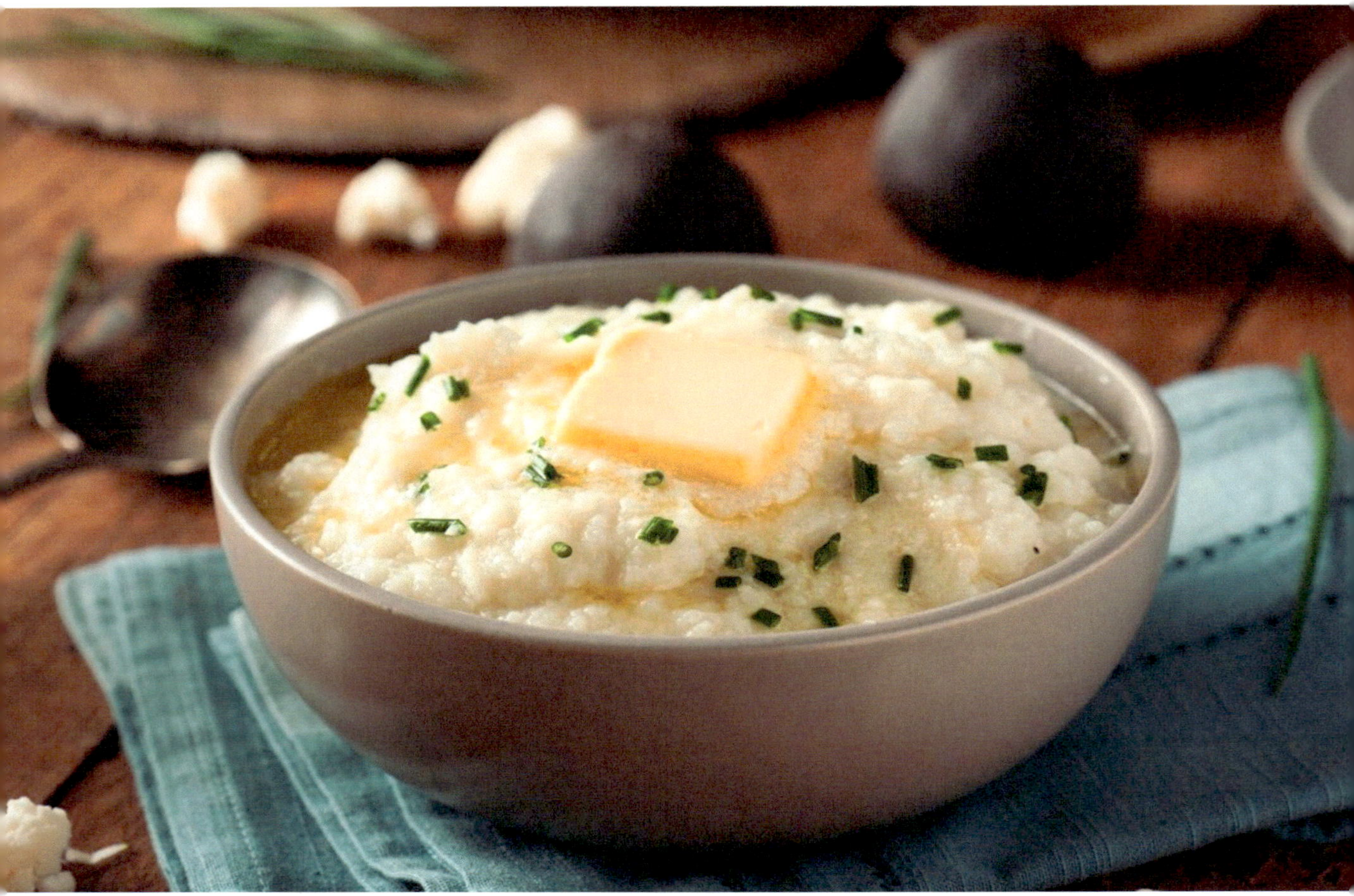

Servings: 6

Ingredients:

1 lb l 450 g cauliflower florets
½ cup chicken or vegetable broth*
1 cup heavy whipping cream**
½ teaspoon garlic powder*
½ cup shredded cheddar cheese* salt and pepper, to taste

Method:

I didn't care for any of the recipes I found online, so I had to experiment until I got it right. I only use fresh cauliflower, and I prefer the pre-washed, bagged florets that you can buy in the produce section of most stores.

1. In a large saucepan, add cauliflower and chicken broth.
2. Cook over medium high heat until broth begins to boil.
3. Cover and let it steam for about 5 minutes, or until cauliflower begins to soften.
4. Remove lid, and as it cooks, break the pieces of cauliflower apart with a fork, wooden spoon or potato masher.
5. As you mash it, the cauliflower will release liquid, too.
6. Continue to mash and cook until all the liquid is gone, then add heavy whipping cream and reduce again until it is nice and creamy and not runny.
7. Take it off the heat and stir in salt, pepper and garlic powder. Stir in the shredded cheese to bind it together.

More serving options (not included in macro count):

Loaded Mashed Cauliflower:

1. Load it up with more shredded cheese, sour cream, bacon bits, and chopped green onion (not included in the macro count).

Cauliflower casserole:

1. Reduce the amount of heavy cream to 1/2 cup

2. After removing the cauliflower mash from the heat, stir in 4 ounces cream cheese, ¼ teaspoon smoked paprika (omit if nightshade intolerant), ½ cup shredded smoked gouda cheese and one teaspoon fresh minced garlic.
3. Spread into a medium casserole dish, top with 1 cup shredded sharp cheddar cheese,
4. ½ cup cooked and crumbled bacon and 3 chopped green onions.
5. Bake at 425 °F/220 °C until cheese is bubbly and browned on top - about 20 minutes.

*Check garlic powder allergen list for gluten. Check shredded cheese and broth allergen list for gluten and check both for nightshades.
**Check cream for emulsifiers and allergen list for gluten.

Gluten free | Egg free | Nut free | Nightshade free | Lacto Vegetarian option

Serving size	Protein	Fat	Total Carbs	Net Carbs
5.1 oz 145 g	5.2 g	17.9 g	5.4 g	3.9 g

The discovery of a new dish
does more for the happiness
of the human race
than the discovery of a star.

~Jean Anthelme Brillat-Savarin,
The Physiology of Taste: Or,
Meditations on Transcendental Gastronomy

Cauliflower - Oven Roasted

Courtesy John Starchman, Red Onion Cafe, Joplin, Missouri

Mende

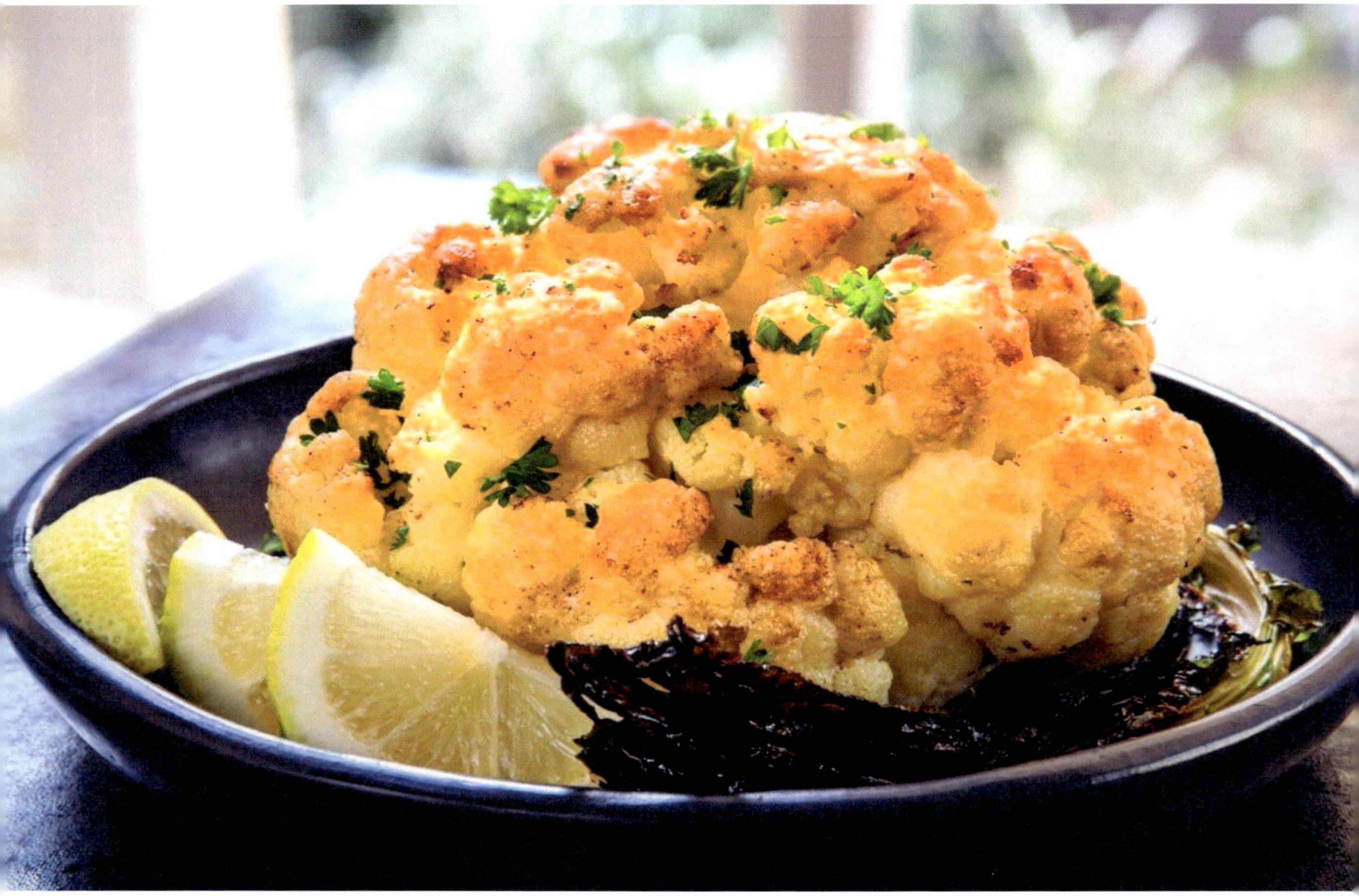

Servings: 6

Ingredients:

1 medium head I approx. 550 g of cauliflower
2 teaspoon red pepper flakes* (omit if nightshade intolerant, or replace with cracked pepper)
1 tablespoon fresh thyme, stalk removed
1 teaspoon granulated garlic (check if gluten free)
1 tablespoon coarse salt 1 stick I 114 g salted butter
2 tablespoon coconut oil
Juice from half a lemon (optional, included in macro count)

Method:

1. Pre-heat oven to 425°F/220°C.
2. Melt the coconut oil and the butter together
3. Put the cauliflower in a large bowl, coat with melted butter and coconut oil.
4. Add dry seasonings, mix together evenly.
5. Place on a tray and bake for 18 minutes, or until the florets are golden brown and crispy, stirring halfway through.
6. Remove from the oven and give it a squeeze of lemon juice, if using.

Gluten free option | Egg free | Nut free | Nightshade free option | Lacto Vegetarian

Serving size	Protein	Fat	Total Carbs	Net Carbs
3.3 oz 93 g	1.4 g	15.2 g	3.4 g	1.7 g

Cheesy Skillet Bread

Mende

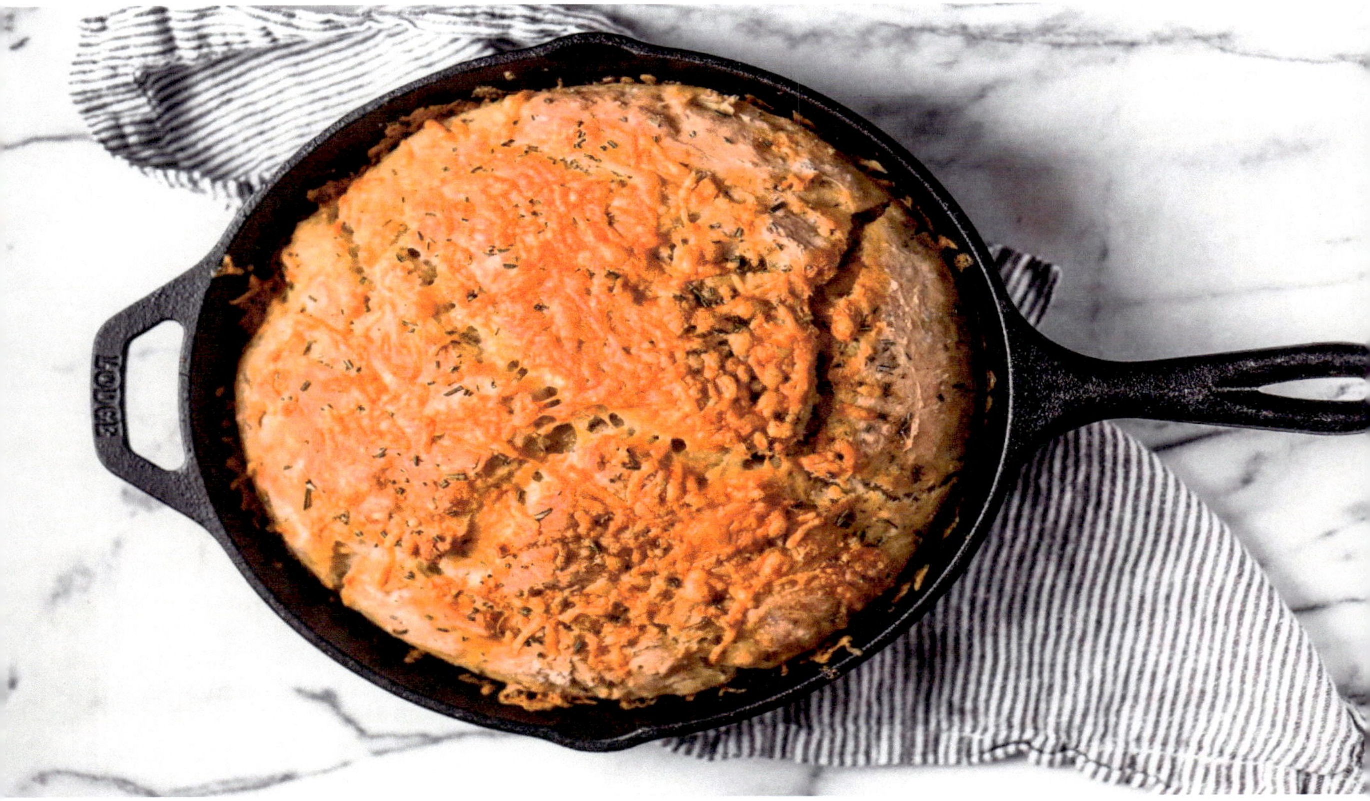

Servings: 8

Ingredients:

1 tablespoon bacon grease or salted butter for the skillet
2 cups almond flour*
½ cup golden flax meal*
2 teaspoon of baking powder (aluminium and gluten free)
½ teaspoon salt
1 ½ cups shredded** sharp cheddar cheese, mozzarella cheese, or smoked gouda cheese, divided
3 large eggs, beaten
½ cup salted butter, melted
¾ cup chicken broth**, almond milk*** or water. Macro count uses broth.

Optional additions:

Fresh minced garlic, fresh chopped herbs, chopped scallions, or your choice of dried herbs and/or spices - not suitable if using recipe for stuffing (and not included in macro count).

Method:

1. Preheat oven to 425°F/220°C.
2. Measure all ingredients and have them ready to assemble.
3. Put the butter in a 10-inch iron skillet and place in the oven until butter is melted and bubbly, but not burned. About 10 minutes.
4. While the skillet is heating, in a large mixing bowl, whisk together almond flour, flax seed meal, baking powder, salt and 1 cup shredded cheddar cheese.
5. Stir in the eggs, melted butter and almond milk until thoroughly combined.
6. Stir in any optional additions but keep it plain if you're planning to turn this into stuffing.
7. Remove hot skillet from oven (don't forget the handle will be hot!), and swirl butter to coat sides.
8. our batter into pan. Sprinkle with remaining cheese.
9. Bake 16 to 20 minutes, or until browned at the edges and set through the middle. Cheese on top should be nicely browned.
10. Remove and let cool 15 minutes.
11. Serve warm with plenty of butter, or reserve for making stuffing.

*Check allergen list for gluten. Check for nightshades.

**Check allergen list for gluten. Check for nightshades such as potato starch and spices.

***Check for vegetable oil, emulsifiers and sugar.

Gluten free | Nightshade free | Lacto/Ovo/Vegetarian

Serving size	Protein	Fat	Total Carbs	Net Carbs
4.2 oz 118 g	15.8 g	38.9 g	10.9 g	3.8 g

...no one is born a great cook,
one learns by doing.
~Julia Child

Cranberry-Strawberry Sauce

Mende

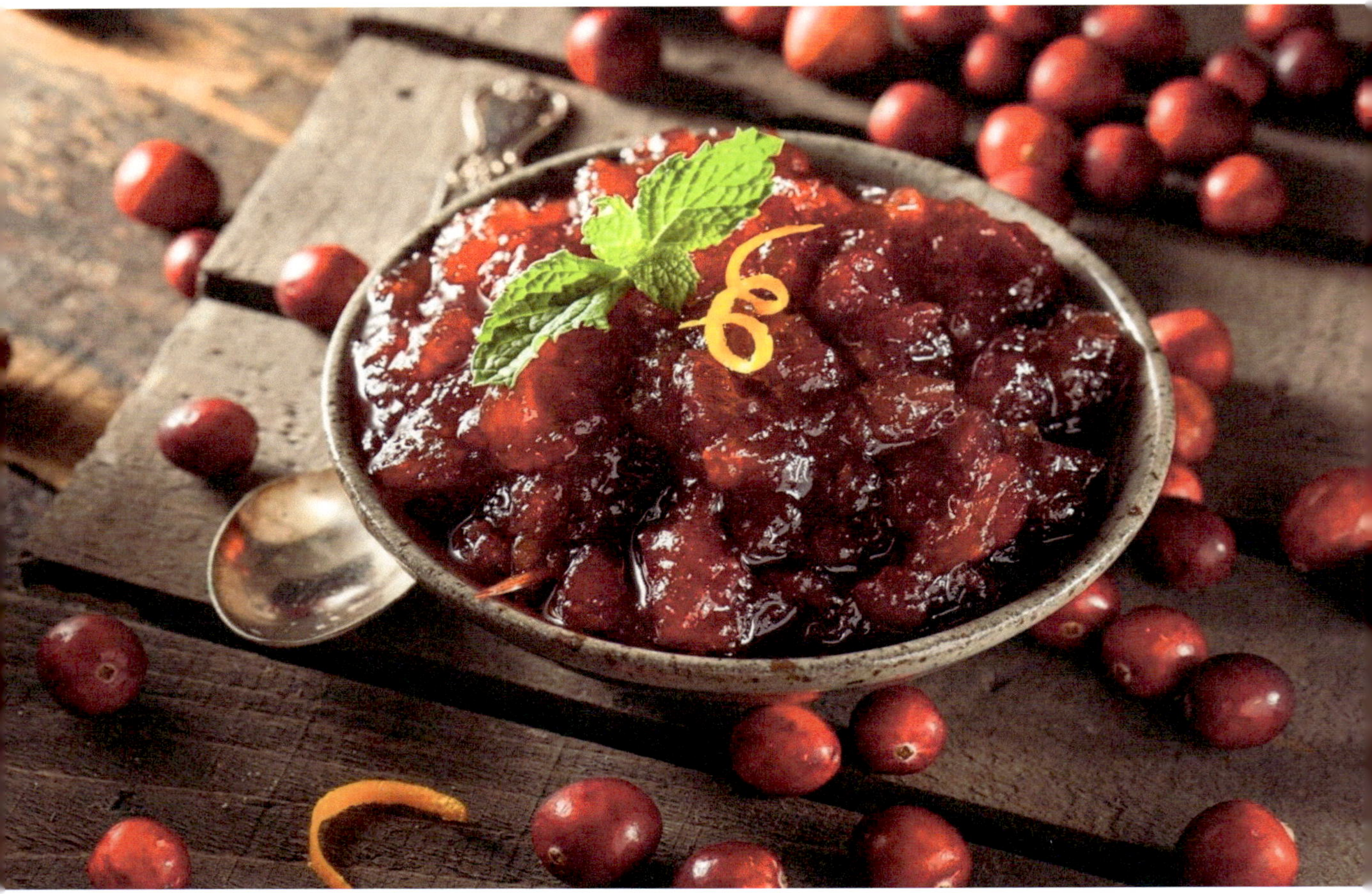

Servings: 72 tablespoons

Ingredients:

3 cups cranberries
1 lb | 450 g package frozen unsweetened strawberries (defrosted and juice saved)
1 cup Gentle Sweet*

Method:

1. Place cranberries with strawberry juice (add water to make ½ cup of liquid, if necessary) in a large, heavy saucepan.
2. Cook over medium to high heat, stirring constantly, until the berries burst and the mixture begins to thicken.
3. Add strawberries and continue to cook the sauce until it's nice and thick, but don't cook too long or the strawberries will turn dull in color.
4. Remove from heat and cool completely before adding the sweetener. Mix well.
5. Serve with roasted turkey, chicken or ham, or add a dollop of whipped cream for a yummy treat.

*Gentle Sweet is a natural, non-caloric sweetener blend of erythritol, xylitol and pure stevia powder. Please be mindful that these sweeteners may still cause increased blood glucose, increased insulin response or inflammatory flare-ups in some individuals.

Gluten free | Egg free | Nut free | Dairy free | Nightshade free | Vegetarian

Serving size	Protein	Fat	Total Carbs	Net Carbs
1 tbsp	0 g	0 g	4.3 g	3.9 g

Green Bean Ketolicious Casserole

Mende

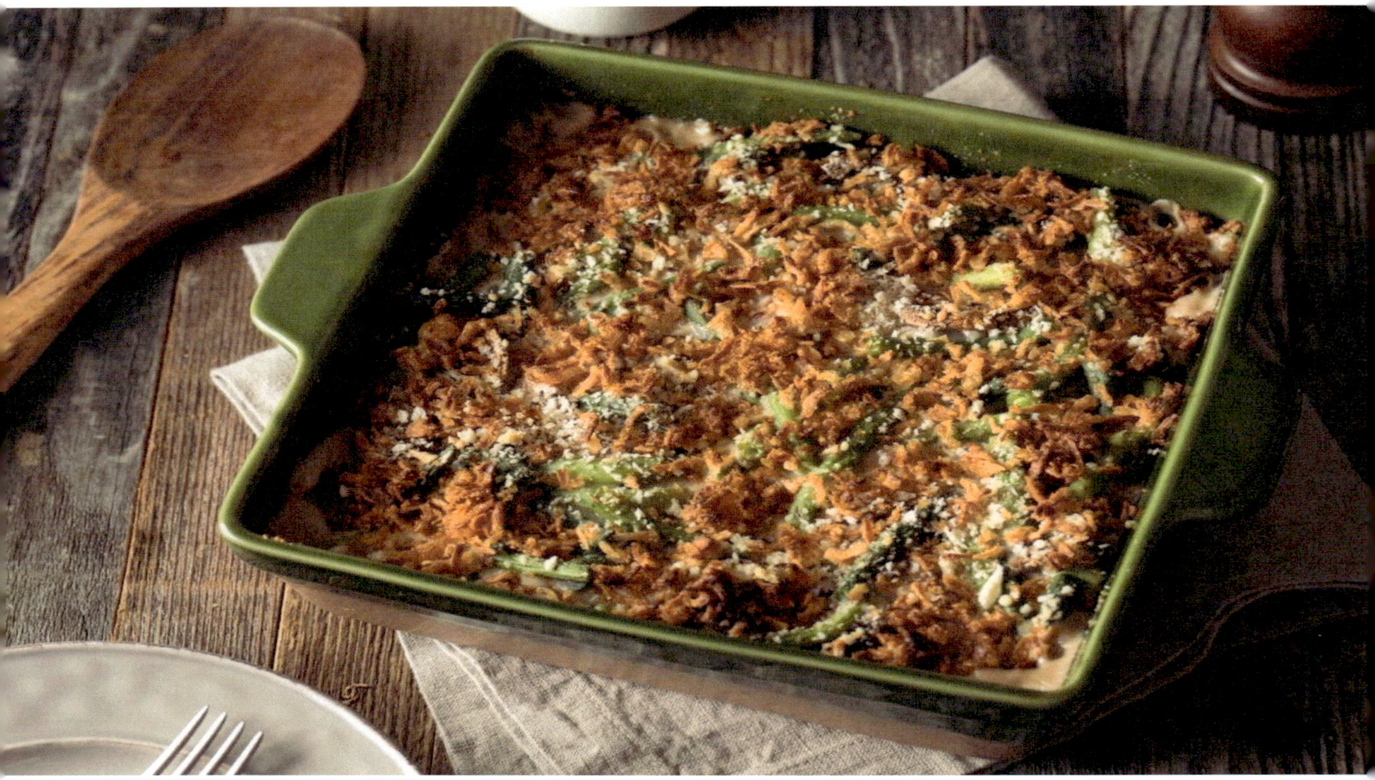

Servings: 10

Ingredients:

1 pound | 450 g frozen or fresh green beans (frozen are preferred)
8 ounces | 220 g sliced mushrooms
1 stick | 114 g real salted butter, divided into 2 portions
½ large onion or one whole small onion, thinly sliced and divided
1 ½ cups heavy whipping cream*
½ cup almond flour**
½ cup dry parmesan cheese***
1 teaspoon salt, or to taste
¼ teaspoon black pepper, or to taste
½ teaspoon garlic powder**

Method:

1. Preheat oven to 425 °F/220 °C.
2. Melt half of the butter in a large, deep skillet over medium heat.
3. Add the green beans and half the sliced onion to the skillet and salt well. Green beans should sizzle when you add them. If not, turn heat up. Allow veggies to cook, stirring only occasionally to allow some caramelization to happen.
4. In a separate skillet over medium heat, melt the other half of the butter and add the rest of the sliced onions and salt. Allow the onions to caramelize in the butter. Stir occasionally to keep the onions from scorching.
5. Once green beans have developed some caramelization, move them to the sides of the pan and add the mushrooms and salt, pepper and garlic powder. Cook and stir until mushrooms are browned and cooked through.
6. Pour in one cup of heavy cream, but reserve the other half cup to add later if necessary. Cook and stir to reduce the cream. It should thicken nicely and sauce should coat the vegetables. If mixture looks too dry, add the other half cup of cream. Taste and adjust seasonings.
7. Pour green bean mixture into a medium casserole dish. Top with caramelized onions and parmesan or almond flour mixture (or use all parmesan if you want to decrease the carb count).
8. Bake until casserole is bubbly and the top is nicely browned.

*Check cream for emulsifiers and allergen list for gluten.

**Check allergen list for gluten.

***If prepackaged, check allergen list for gluten, and check for potato starch for nightshade intolerance.

Gluten free options | Egg free | Nut free (optional) |
Nightshade free | Lacto Vegetarian

Serving size	Protein	Fat	Total Carbs	Net Carbs
4.7 oz 133 g	5.2 g	26.4 g	7.3 g	5 g

Holiday Slaw

Raeann

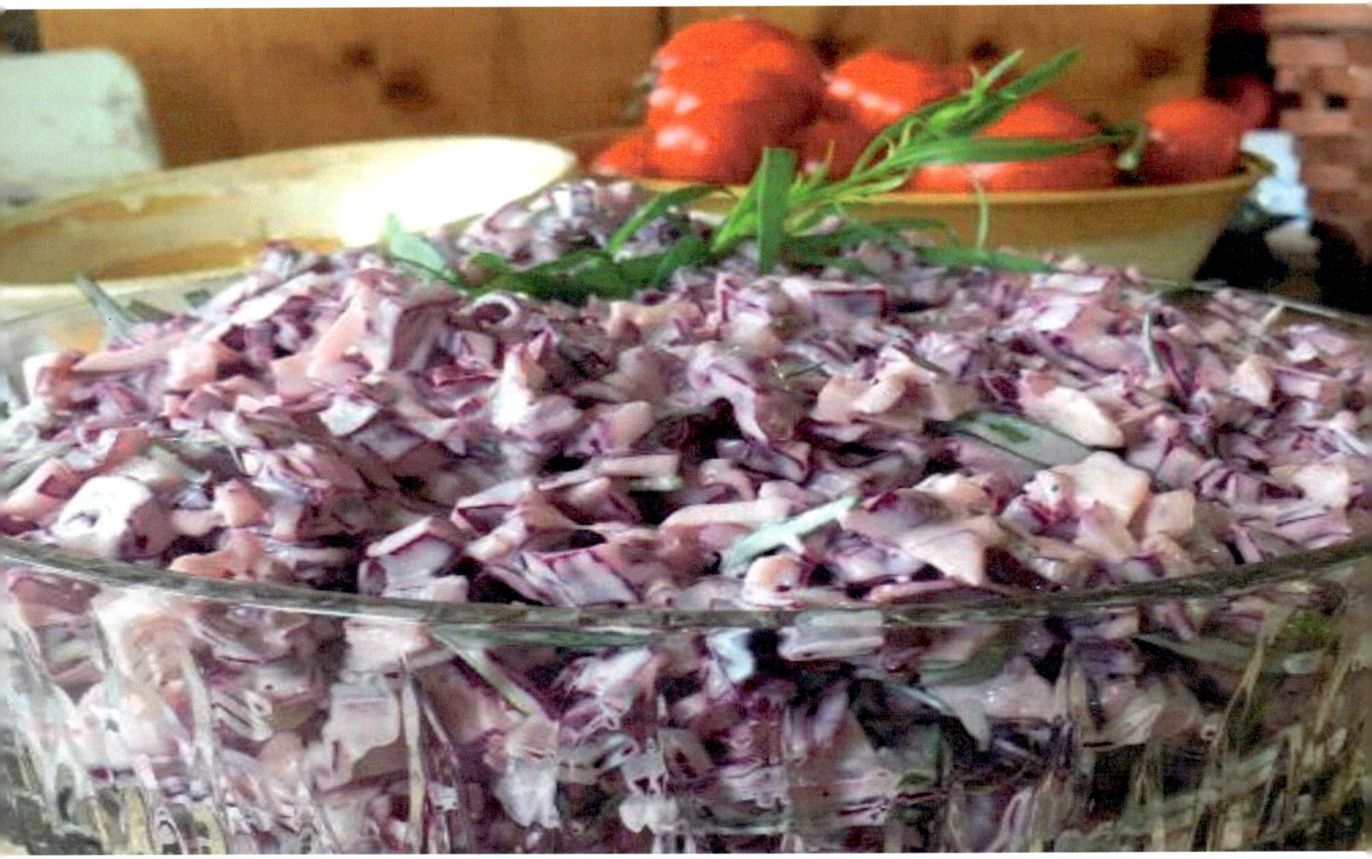

photo courtesy of Raeann Sparks

Servings: 20

Ingredients:

1 large head red cabbage, finely chopped
1 small red onion, finely chopped
3 tablespoon fresh tarragon, or to taste
1 cup sour cream*
1 teaspoon natural salt
¼ teaspoon black pepper
3 drops pure stevia extract
3 tablespoon apple cider vinegar (ACV)

Method:

1. Mix cabbage, onion and tarragon together in a large bowl.
2. Mix the sour cream, ACV, stevia (try adding a drop at a time, or leave out altogether), salt, and pepper together in a separate bowl. Taste and adjust.
3. Combine all ingredients into one bowl.
4. Refrigerate for at least one hour before serving, to mingle the flavors.

TIP: Make this a day ahead of time and it's even better.

*Check sour cream for emulsifiers and check allergen list for gluten.

Gluten free option | Egg free | Nut free | Nightshade free | Lacto Vegetarian

Serving size	Protein	Fat	Total Carbs	Net Carbs
2.6 oz 75 g	1.2 g	2.3 g	5.2 g	3.9 g

Skillet Fried Green Vegetables with Mushroom Sauce

(shown with green beans)

Mende

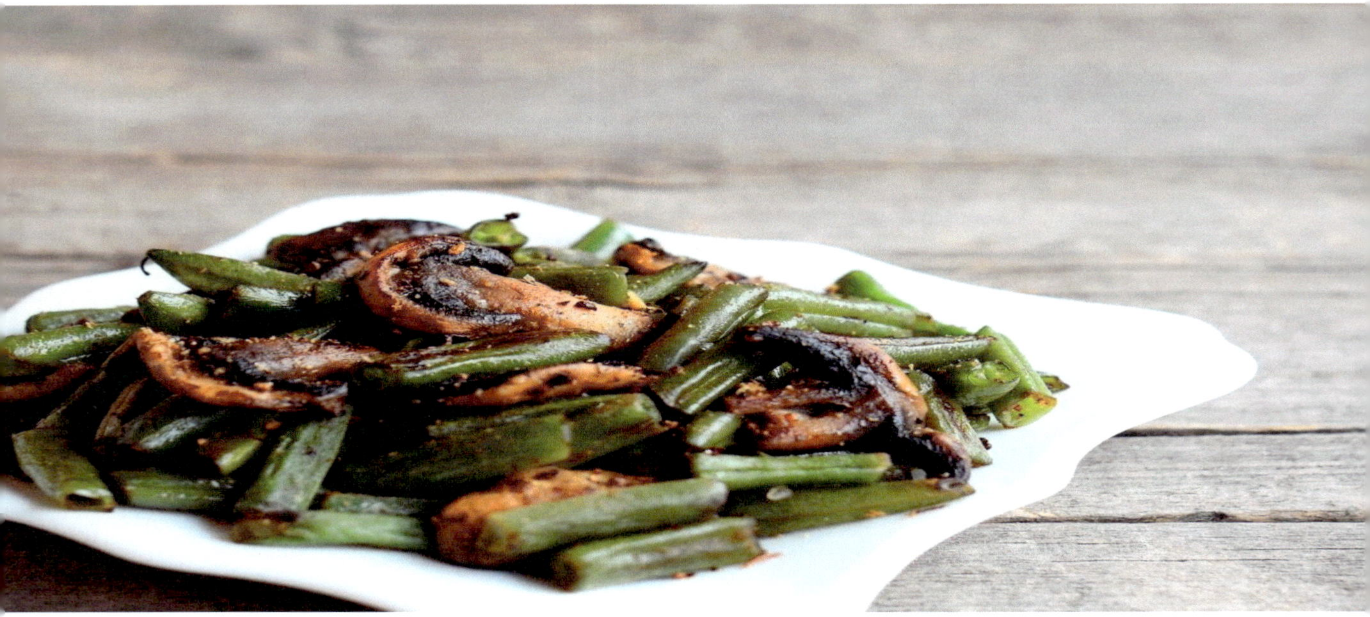

Servings: 4

Ingredients:

½ stick | 55 g salted butter (or ½ cup extra virgin olive oil or coconut oil for dairy free)
1 slice bacon*, chopped or whole (omit for vegetarian)
¼ medium onion, slivered or chopped
2 cloves garlic, smashed or minced (optional)
1 pound | 450 g fresh or frozen green vegetables of your choice: green beans, asparagus, broccoli, sliced zucchini, brussel sprouts, mushrooms or combine to taste
¼ teaspoon garlic powder*
Salt and pepper, to taste

Method:

1. Melt the butter in a 12-inch diameter deep skillet with a lid.
2. Add onion and bacon. Cook over medium-low heat until onion is tender and bacon is rendered but not crispy.
3. Add the garlic and cook for an additional minute or so. Raise heat to medium and cook until the onions begin to caramelize.
4. Add green veggies all at once. They should sizzle when you add them. Season with salt, pepper, and garlic powder. Cook as you toss the veggies in the butter until they begin to caramelize slightly. Add in mushrooms.
5. Reduce heat to low, cover skillet with a lid and continue to cook for another 15-20 minutes or until veggies are tender. Adjust seasonings before serving.

Macro note: Macro count based on using green beans.

*Check for bacon allergen list for gluten, check for spices if nightshade intolerant. Check garlic powder allergen list for gluten.

Gluten free option | Egg free | Nut free | Dairy Free option
Nightshade free option | Lacto Vegetarian option

Serving size	Protein	Fat	Total Carbs	Net Carbs
3.2 oz. 91 g	2.1 g	8.1 g	6.8 g	4.3 g

Wilted Spinach with Bacon and Onions

Courtesy John Starchman, Red Onion Cafe, Joplin, Missouri

Mende

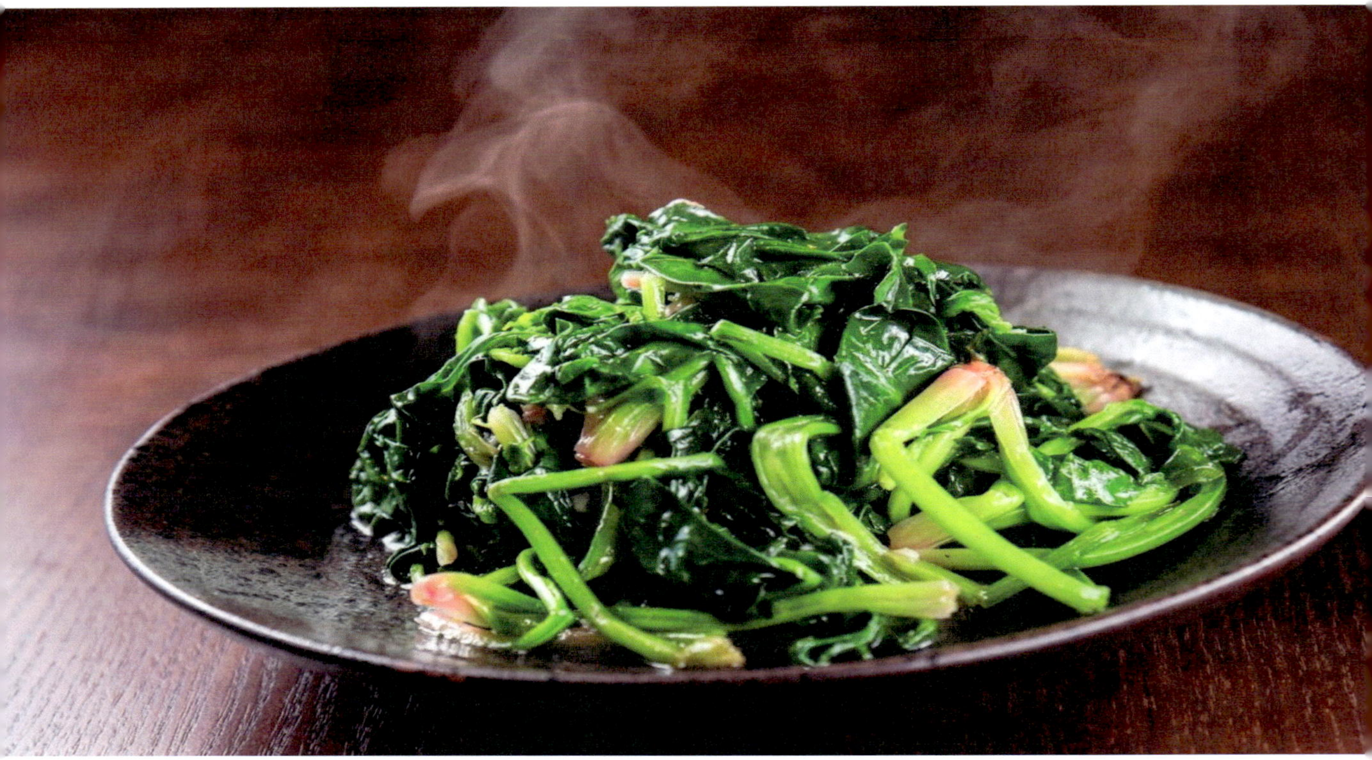

Servings: 4

Ingredients:

4 strips bacon*, chopped
4 cups spinach
¼ cup green onions, chopped
¼ teaspoon red pepper flakes*, optional (omit if nightshade intolerant)
¼ teaspoon granulated garlic*
1 tablespoon white wine vinegar OR lemon juice
Salt & black pepper, to taste

Note: Check herbs and spices for gluten, check bacon for gluten and spices if nightshade intolerant.

Method:

1. Cook the bacon until rendered.
2. Add green onions and add them to the bacon, toss to coat in the bacon grease.
3. Add the spinach to the pan, and quickly add the rest of your seasonings, and stir. It will reduce in volume significantly.
4. As soon as the spinach has wilted, give it a splash of white wine vinegar or lemon juice, and serve warm.

Variation: Omit the vinegar or lemon juice, substitute with a splash of heavy cream**, and make creamed spinach (not included in macro count).

*Check bacon allergen list for gluten. Check herbs and spices allergen list for gluten.
**Check cream for emulsifiers, and allergen list for gluten.

Gluten free option | Egg free | Nut free | Dairy free option | Nightshade free option

Serving size	Protein	Fat	Total Carbs	Net Carbs
1.5 oz. 43 g	3.6 g	2.9 g	1.6 g	0.9 g

Pull up a chair.

Take a taste.

Come join us.

Life is so endlessly delicious.

~Ruth Reichl

Desserts

"You are how you eat. How you eat has more to do with tasting things carefully. When you taste something, do you taste the earth, the sky, the sunlight and the water? Do you taste the effort and work of other people in the growing and preparation of the food? Is there any sense of thanks, appreciation or gratitude?"

~Edward Espe Brown

Chocolate Pecan Torte

Mende

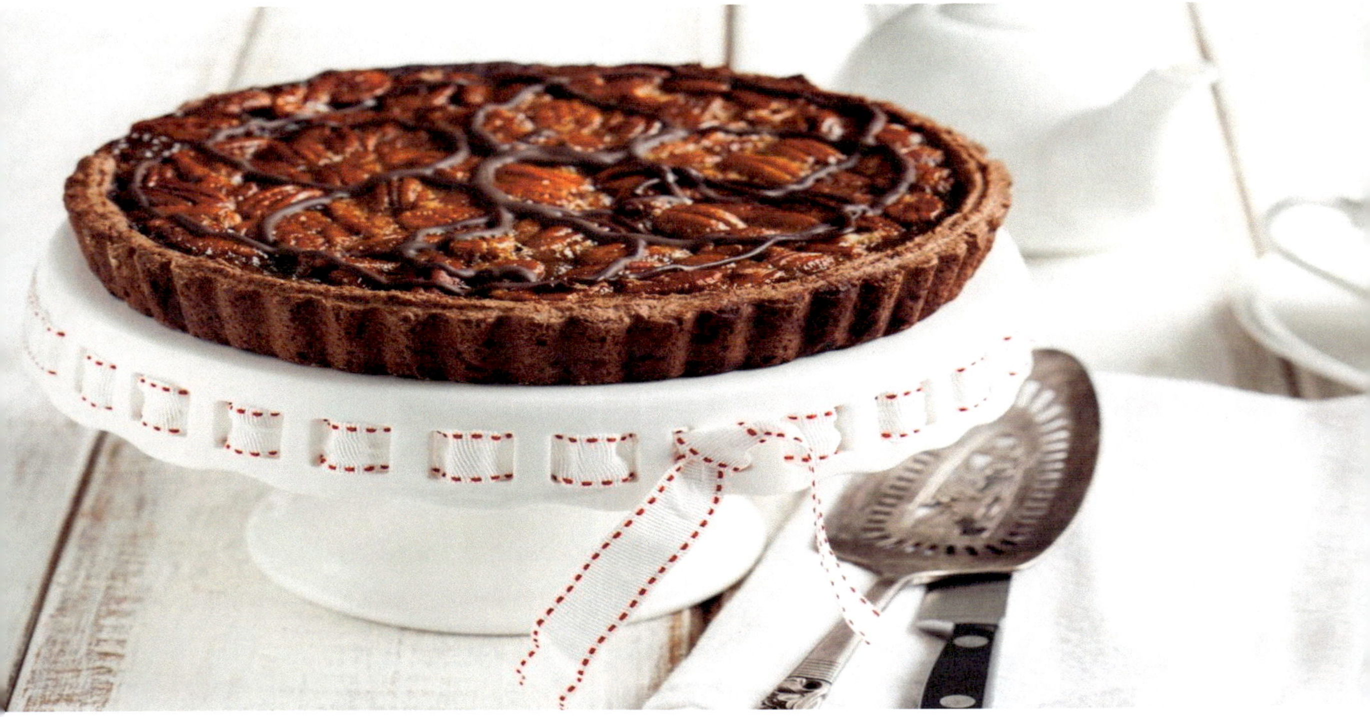

Servings: 16

Ingredients:

4 oz. (one bar) | 112 g Baker's unsweetened baking chocolate, broken into pieces
2 sticks | 228 g salted butter
A little extra butter or lard (use butter if lacto vegetarian) for greasing
1 ½ cups Gentle Sweet*
1 teaspoon Goodman's vanilla, or vanilla extract or flavoring (no sugar)
6 large eggs, at room temperature
½ cup unsweetened cocoa or raw cacao powder
1 ½ cups pecan halves or pieces
¼ teaspoon salt

Method:

1. Preheat the oven to 325 °F/160 °C.
2. Lightly grease (with lard or butter) a 9-inch round pan. Line the bottom of the pan with parchment paper and grease the paper, too.
3. Heat the chocolate and the butter together in a microwave-safe bowl until butter and chocolate are both melted. It's best to heat for 1 minute, stir, then 30 seconds and stir, etc. to avoid spoiling the taste of the chocolate, until the chocolate is completely melted.
4. In the bowl of a stand mixer, or in a large mixing bowl, beat eggs until foamy.
5. Add Gentle Sweet and beat until mixture is light and lemony in color.
6. Beat in vanilla, salt and cocoa powder.
7. While mixer is running, gradually pour the melted chocolate/butter mixture into the eggs in a thin stream.
8. Continue to beat an additional minute.
9. Stir in pecans.
10. Pour into prepared pan.
11. Bake 20-25 minutes until edges are set but the center is still jiggly.
12. Chill before serving.

*Gentle Sweet is a natural, non-caloric sweetener blend of erythritol, xylitol and pure stevia powder. Please be mindful that these sweeteners may still cause increased blood glucose, increased insulin response or inflammatory flare-ups in some individuals.

Gluten free option | Nightshade free | Lacto Vegetarian option

This decadent dessert has a high total carbohydrate content because it contains sugar alcohols. Erythritol is not counted as a carb as it is not digested, and xylitol is only counted as 50% carbs as it is only partly digested, therefore significantly lowering the net carbs. It is a dessert to eat in small quantities infrequently.

Serving size	Protein	Fat	Total Carbs	Net Carbs
2.5 oz 72 g	4.7 g	25 g	26.9 g	11.1 g

Merry Christmas

&

Ketolicious New Year

Cream Cheese Whipped Cream

Mende

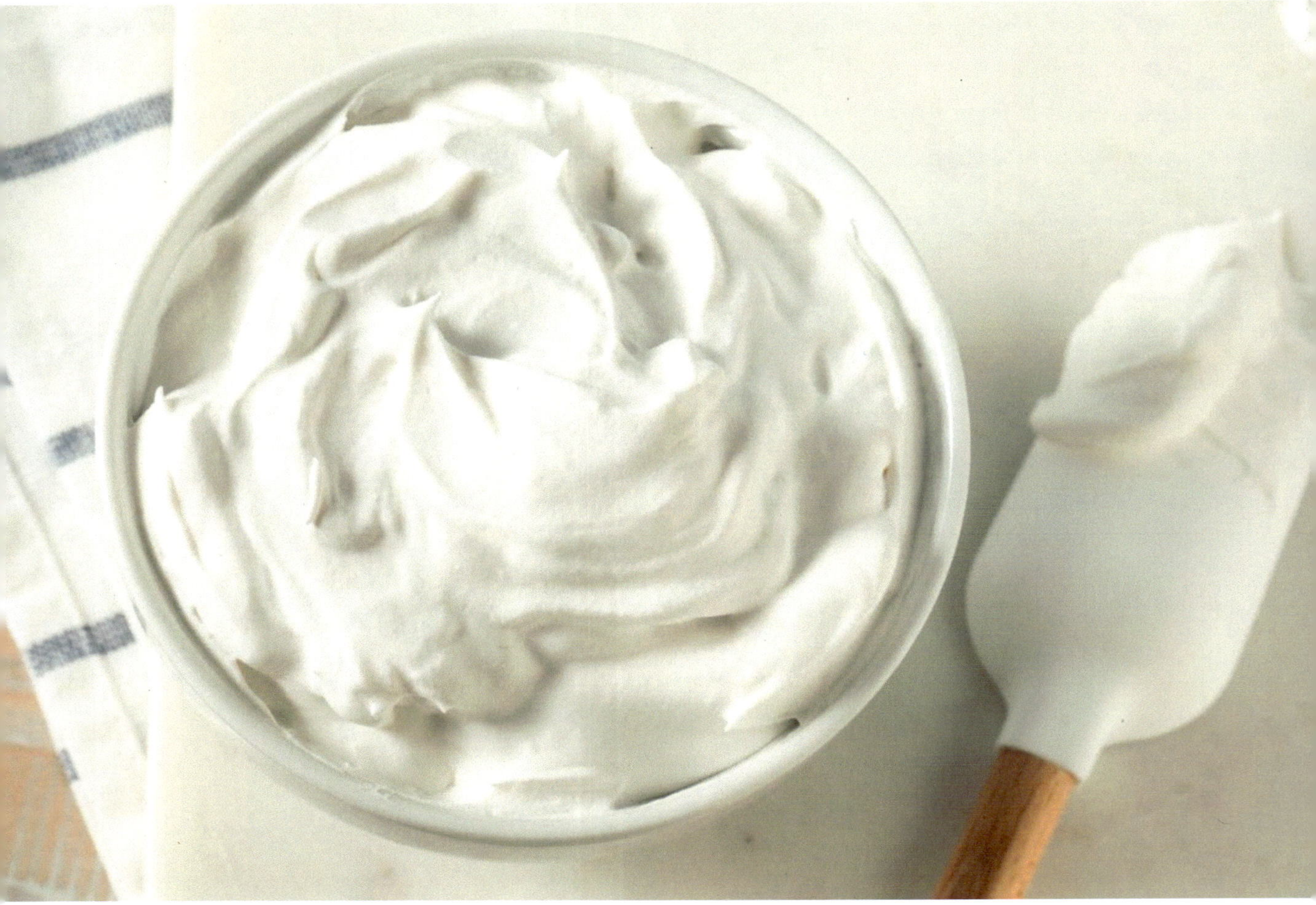

Servings: 8

Ingredients:

16 oz. | 450 g of cream cheese*, cold
2 cups of heavy whipping cream*
2 teaspoon vanilla or lemon extract (check gluten free)
8 packets | 8 g of stevia, or to taste

Method:

1. Beat cold cream cheese in an electric mixer until it begins to soften. Do not let it get warm.
2. Add about a half cup of the heavy whipping cream and beat until mixture is thickened and fluffy. Do not overbeat.
3. Add another half cup of cream and beat. Continue adding and beating until mixture reaches the desired consistency and will hold a stiff peak.
4. Stir in vanilla and sweetener.

Serving suggestions:

Layer the filling with fresh sliced strawberries.

Use as a filling for cream cheese keto crepes.

This also works as a dip for berries or frosting for cake.

Note: Variations not included in macro count.

*Check cream and cream cheese for emulsifiers and allergen list for gluten.

Gluten free option | Egg free | Nut free | Nightshade free | Lacto Vegetarian

Serving size	Protein	Fat	Total Carbs	Net Carbs
4.2 oz. 118 g	5.1 g	40.8 g	5.7 g	5.7 g

Creme Brulee (Egg Custard)

Mende

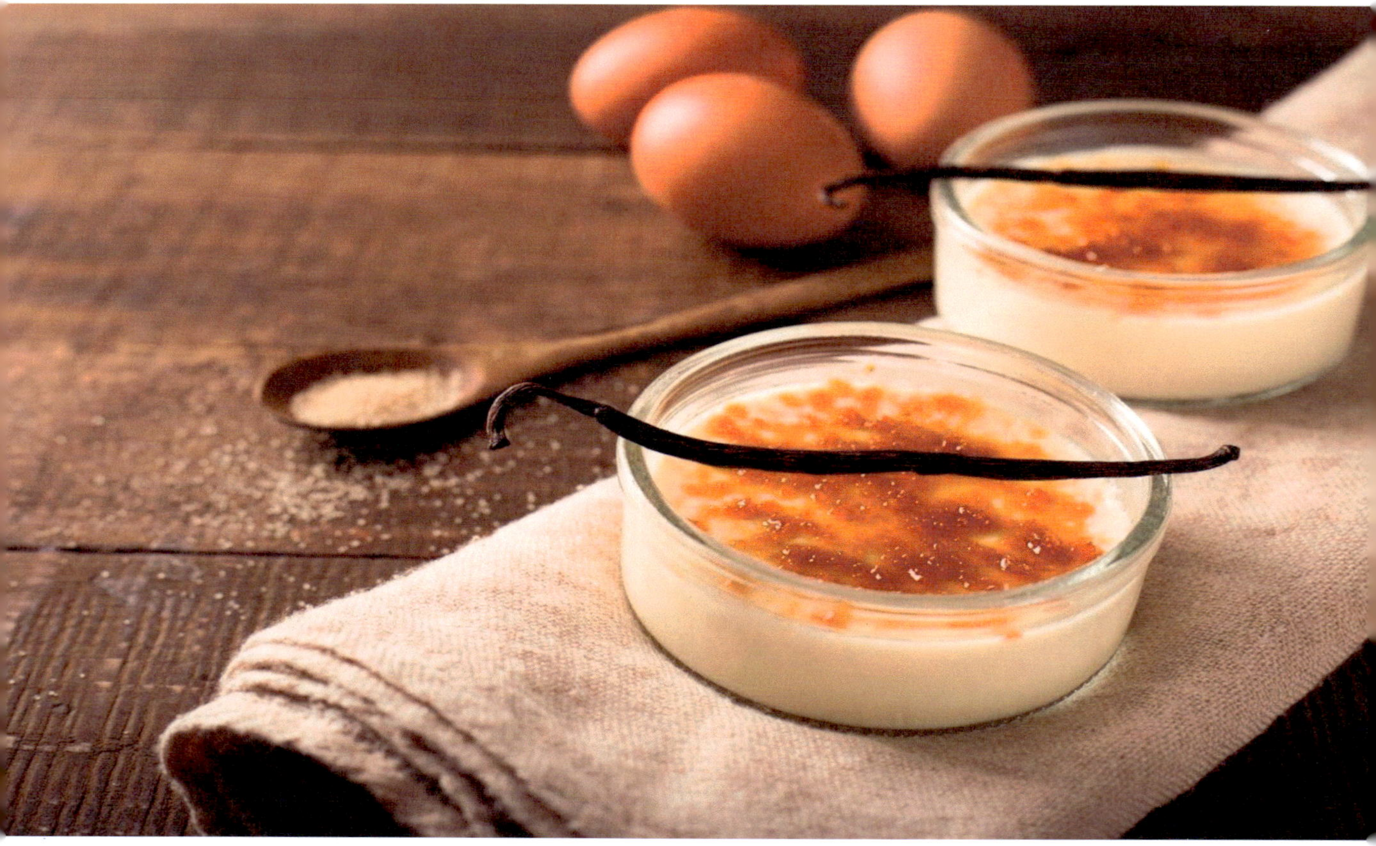

Servings: 8

Ingredients:

3 cups heavy whipping cream*
6 egg yolks, beaten
½ cup Gentle Sweet** plus 6 tablespoons | 187 g
1 vanilla bean, sliced opened and contents scraped
¼ teaspoon salt
1 teaspoon Goodman's Vanilla, or 1 teaspoon vanilla extract or flavoring (no sugar)
1 tablespoon butter, melted

Method:

1. Preheat the oven to 350 °F/ 175 °C.
2. Heat the heavy cream with ½ cup Gentle Sweet, vanilla bean pod and scrapings, salt and Goodman's vanilla or vanilla extract.
3. Remove from heat and remove and discard vanilla bean pod.
4. Gradually beat about ½ cup of the hot cream into the egg yolks. Slowly stir the tempered yolks into the pan with the cream.
5. Set 6 ramekins into a large baking dish. Pour hot water in the dish around the ramekins to come halfway up the sides.
6. Carefully ladle the liquid custard into the ramekins.
7. Bake for 30 minutes, or until custard is just set on the edges and jiggly in the middle.
8. Remove the ramekins from the water bath and chill until custard is set.
9. Combine melted butter with the reserved 6 tablespoons of Gentle Sweet.
10. Sprinkle 1 tablespoon sweetener mixture on each of the custards.
11. With a blow torch or under the broiler, caramelize the sweetener mixture to create a candy shell. Serve once the candy is cooled and crunchy.

*Check cream for emulsifiers, and allergen list for gluten.

**Gentle Sweet is a natural, non-caloric sweetener blend of erythritol, xylitol and pure stevia powder. Please be mindful that these sweeteners may still cause increased blood glucose, increased insulin response or inflammatory flare-ups in some individuals.

Gluten free | Nut free | Nightshade free | Lacto Vegetarian

This decadent dessert has a high total carbohydrate content because it contains sugar alcohols. Erythritol is not counted as a carb as it is not digested, and xylitol is only counted as 50% carbs as it is only partly digested, therefore significantly lowering the net carbs. It is a dessert to eat in small quantities infrequently.

Serving size	Protein	Fat	Total Carbs	Net Carbs
4.4 oz 126 g	4.3 g	36.5 g	29.6 g	13.3 g

May your season be full of wonder

&

Luxurious delicious

Ketolicious food too!

Pumpkin Pie with Pecans

Mende

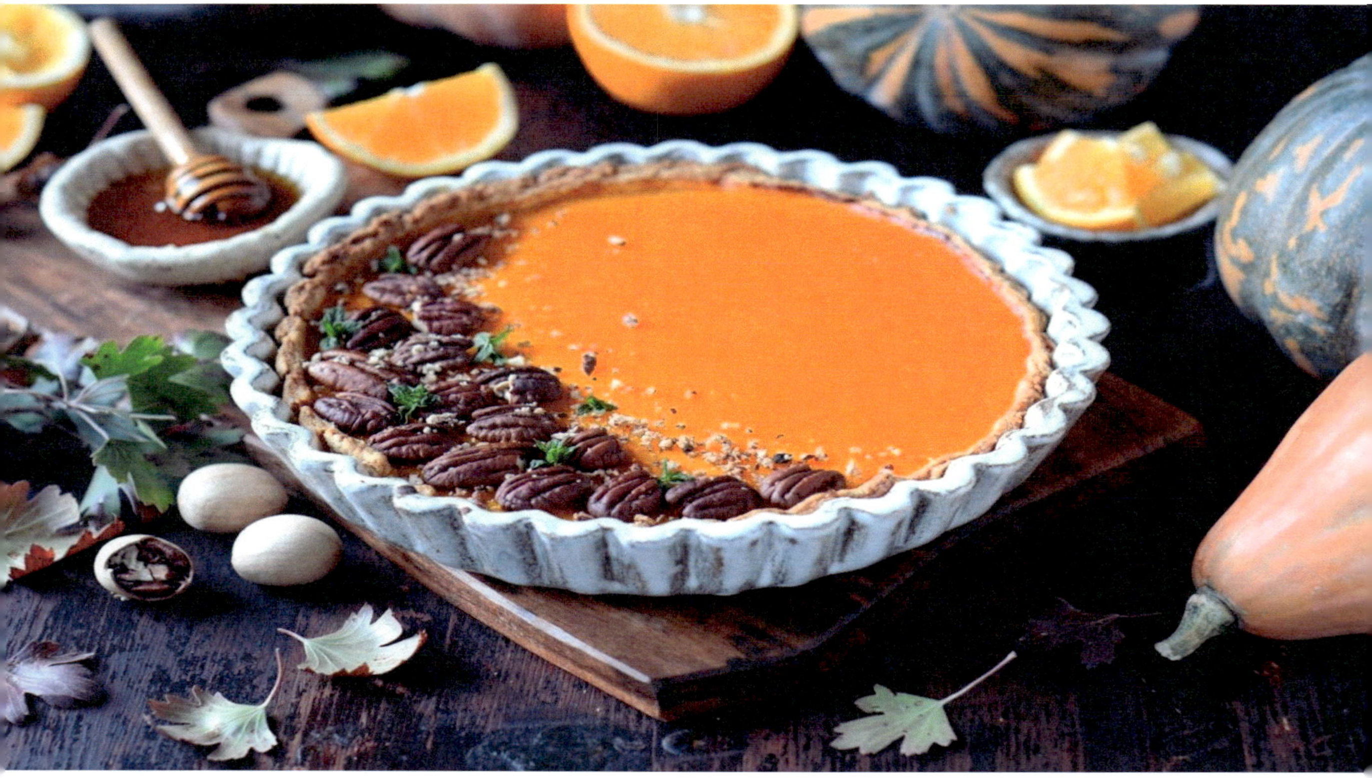

Servings: 8

Ingredients:

1 x Mende's Favorite Low-Carb Pie Crust, cooked as per instructions
1 x 15-oz. | 420 g can pumpkin puree, or 2 cups cooked, pureed and drained fresh pumpkin or butternut squash
1 ½ cups heavy whipping cream 2 eggs, well beaten
¾ cup Gentle Sweet* OR ¾ teaspoon pure Stevia Powder if intolerant to sugar alcohols
½ teaspoon salt
2 teaspoon ground Saigon cinnamon (or other good quality cinnamon)
½ teaspoon ground ginger
¼ teaspoon ground cloves

¼ to ½ teaspoon freshly grated nutmeg
1 tablespoon Goodman's vanilla, or vanilla extract, or vanilla flavoring (no sugar)
½ pecans for decoration (optional)

Method:

1. Preheat the oven to 325° F/160° C.
2. Stir to combine all ingredients except the cream.
3. Gradually stir in the cream.
4. Pour into prepared crust and bake for 45 minutes to an hour, or until the edges are set and center is still slightly jiggly.
5. Cool then refrigerate. You won't need additional whipped cream.

Gluten free | Nut free | Nightshade free | Lacto Vegetarian

This decadent dessert has a high total carbohydrate content because it contains sugar alcohols. Erythritol is not counted as a carb as it is not digested, and xylitol is only counted as 50% carbs as it is only partly digested, therefore significantly lowering the net carbs. It is a dessert to eat in small quantities infrequently.

Serving size	Protein	Fat	Total Carbs	Net Carbs
2.8 oz 81 g	2.7 g	20.2 g	15.7 g	12.25 g

Mende's Favorite Low-carb Pie Crust

Servings: 8

Ingredients:

2 cups pecan meal or almond flour
½ stick | 55 g real salted butter, melted
½ teaspoon salt

Optional ingredients:

¼ cup Splenda or equivalent
½ teaspoon baking powder, (gluten and aluminium free)
1 tablespoon Goodman's vanilla, or vanilla extract, or vanilla flavor (no sugar)
Optional ingredients not included in macro count.

Method:

1. Preheat oven to 350° F/175° C.
2. Combine all ingredients in a bowl and mix well.
3. Work dough with your hands to make sure all the butter is mixed well with the nut meal.
4. Press into a greased pie dish and bake for 10 minutes, or until lightly golden.

TIP: To make your own pecan meal, grind pecans in a food processor until the size of crumbs.

*Gentle Sweet is a natural, non-caloric sweetener blend of erythritol, xylitol and pure stevia powder. Please be mindful that these sweeteners may still cause increased blood glucose, increased insulin response or inflammatory flare-ups in some individuals.

Gluten free option | Egg free | Nightshade free | Lacto Vegetarian

Serving size	Protein	Fat	Total Carbs	Net Carbs
1.1 oz. 31 g	2.2 g	22.8 g	3.3 g	1 g

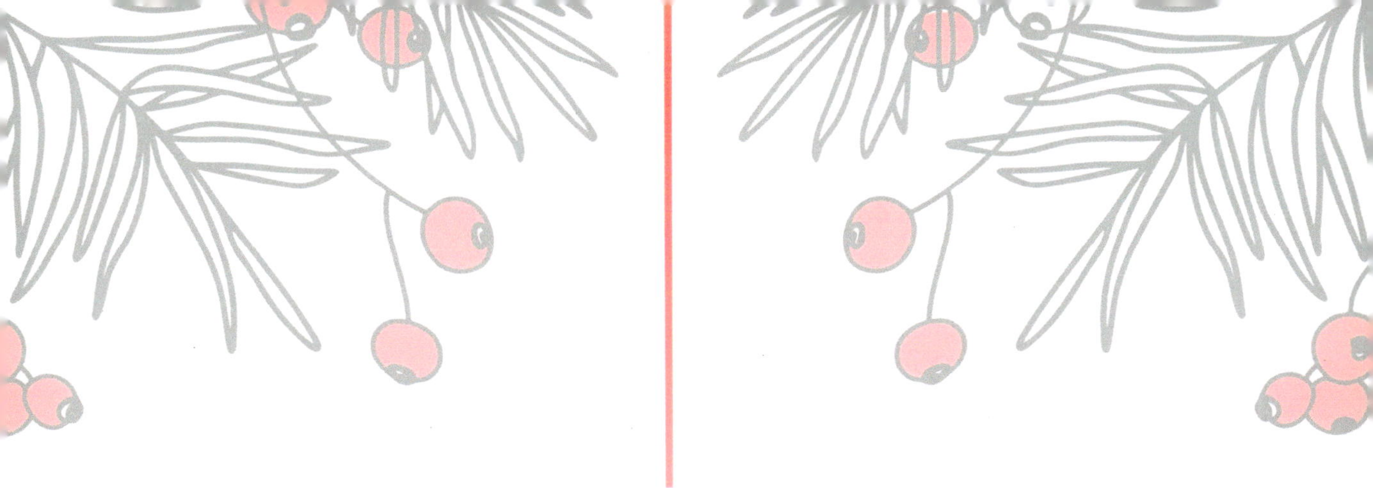

Merry & Bright

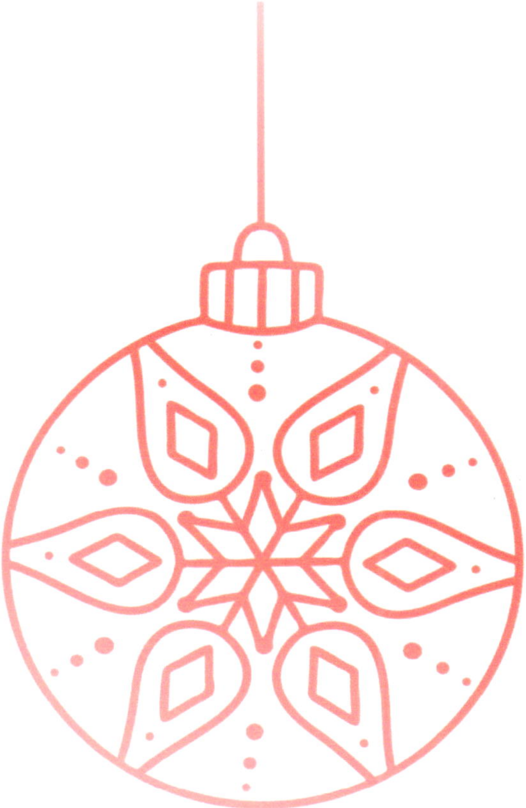

Whipped Cheesecake with Berries

Mende

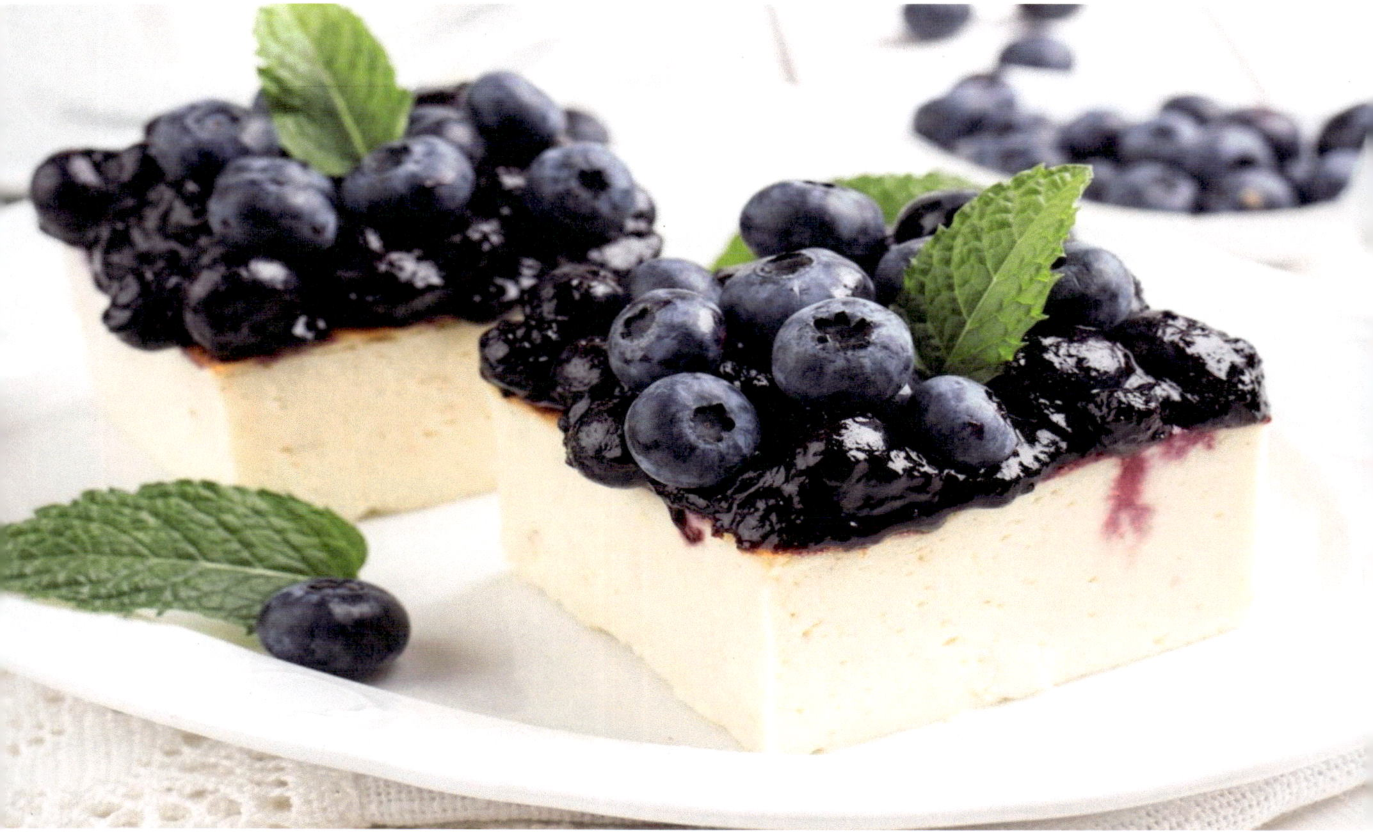

Servings: 12

Ingredients:

"Graham cracker" crust (see recipe below)

Whipped cream cheese filling:

16 ounces | 450 g of cream cheese*
2 cups of heavy whipping cream*
2 teaspoons vanilla or lemon extract
½ cup of monk fruit, or 1/2 cup confectioner's Swerve

Method:

1. Beat cold cream cheese in an electric mixer until it begins to soften. Do not let it get warm.
2. Add about a half cup of cream and beat until mixture is thickened and fluffy. Do not overbeat.
3. Add another half cup of cream and beat. Continue adding and beating until mixture reaches the desired consistency and will hold a stiff peak.
4. Stir in vanilla and sweeten with your preferred sweetener to taste.
5. Spoon into cooled crust and top with fresh berries.

"Graham cracker" Crust

Serves: 12

Ingredients:

½ stick | 55 g salted butter, melted
¼ cup golden flax meal
¼ cup almond flour
¼ cup coconut flour
¼ cup Swerve brown
½ teaspoon vanilla extract
pinch of salt
dash of cinnamon

Note: Check vanilla extract and cinnamon for gluten

Method:

1. Preheat oven to 350 °F/175 °C.
2. Combine all ingredients, press into the bottom of a greased or lined 9 inch pie dish or springform pan.
3. Bake for 10 minutes, or until lightly browned.
4. Cool completely.

*Gentle Sweet is a natural, non-caloric sweetener blend of erythritol, xylitol and pure stevia powder. Please be mindful that these sweeteners may still cause increased blood glucose, increased insulin response or inflammatory flare-ups in some individuals.
*Check cream and cream cheese for emulsifiers and check allergen list for gluten.

Gluten free option | Egg free | Nightshade free | Lacto Vegetarian

Serving size	Protein	Fat	Total Carbs	Net Carbs
2.7 oz 76 g	3.7 g	25.2 g	11.6 g	10.5 g

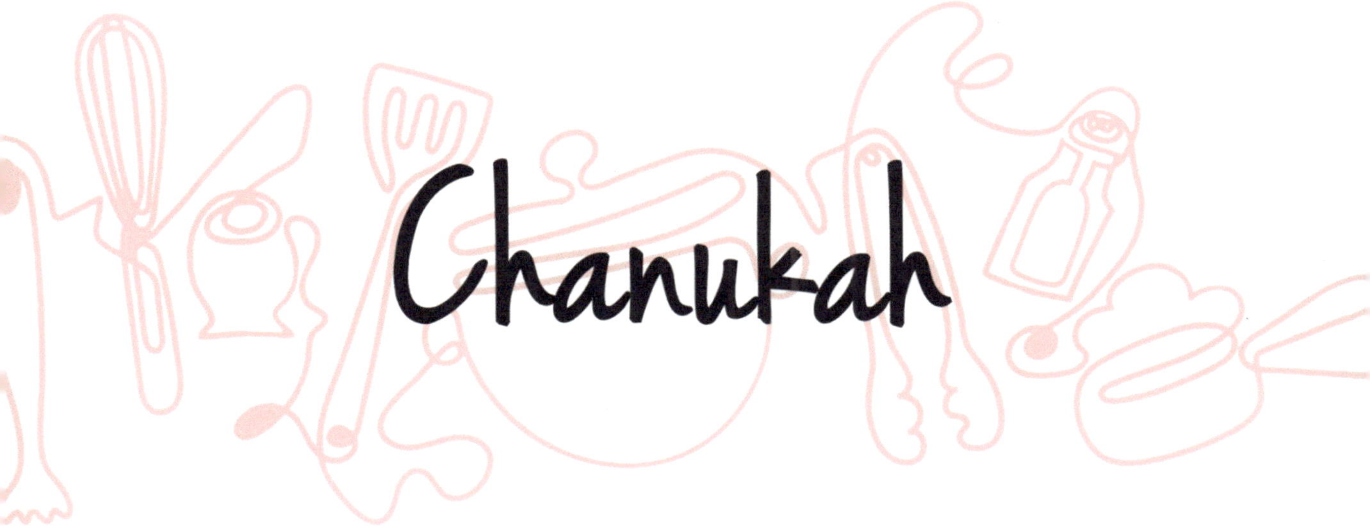

Chanukah

"Waking up is something we can do any time and food is something we do every day. It's such a good time to practice this intention, to be more awake and receive the experience that exists in our hearts."

~Edward Espe Brown

Chanukah – Oil and Light

Brenda

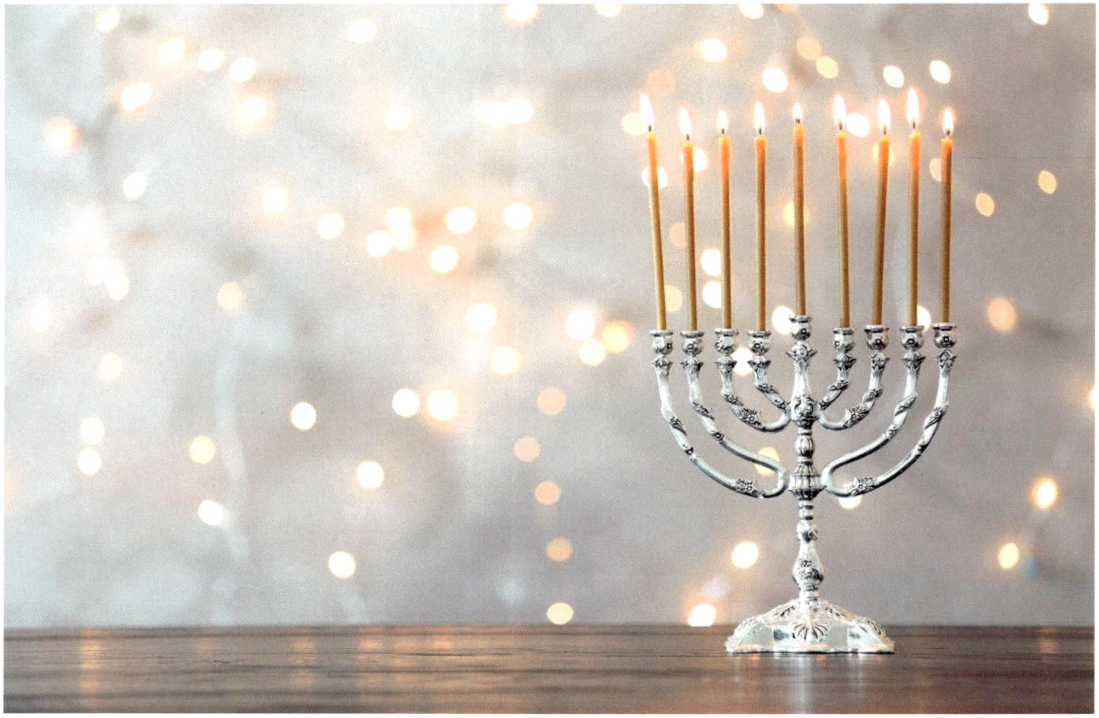

Jewish holiday foods are not just family tradition and comfort - although they are that - or just carefully chosen, combined and prepared ingredients - and here again, they most certainly are - but they are foods and ingredients with history, story, and meaning. Chanukah's quintessential meaningful ingredient is oil - oil because oil was burned to make light in the lamps of the temple in Jerusalem. We use oil consciously for 8 days to honor the memory of the miracle that allowed only one day's worth of lamp oil - (all that was left after a Jewish army retook Jerusalem and the temple following an enemy invasion) - to miraculously last for the eight days it took to prepare the ritually perfect oil for the lamps of the temple.

So oil it is - for eight days. Pan-fried, deep-fried in oil is the preferred cooking method - and of course, the lighting of the eight lights of Chanukah to remind us of - you guessed it oil and light.

Chanukah and Keto

Chanukah has had a bad rap over the last 50 years with the vilification of oil and fats. Over that time some of us were subjected to the indignity of baked potato latkes – tasteless and bland with no oil due to the prevailing fat phobia - all in the name of protecting our health. It became almost an embarrassment to have a holiday dedicated to honoring fat. Chanukah had become politically and dietarily incorrect! But today, we have been liberated by the keto movement to have our fat and oil back to center stage of the Chanukah celebration without shame.

Now that we know better, we can go back to freely celebrating oil and light.

But what about the potato latke which some of us have made synonymous with Chanukah? Of course, the potato was not in the Bible or in the historical records as it was only introduced into Europe and the Middle East after the European invasion and colonization of the Americas. As a part of Jewish Chanukah cuisine, it only dates back to the 1800s in Eastern Europe and was introduced after famine and poverty when vegetable oils were hard to get and potatoes were introduced as a failsafe crop. As you all know by now, potatoes are not keto. What to do now about the Chanukah latke? Well a latke is not a potato. There were lots of latkes before potatoes. The most prized latke was a cheese latke originating in the Italian Jewish community in the middle ages. But we can now make latkes with any low carb veggie. As long as they are cooked in the right kind of good fat or oil, we are all good.

So here is a selection of tried (and loved?) latke recipes that will take you right through the eight days and nights of the celebration of oil and light. Keto friendly and joyous!

Happy Chanukah!

Brenda

Brenda Gold, BHSc (PT)
Lipedema Simplified Coach
brenda@lipedema-simplified.org

Happy

Chanukah

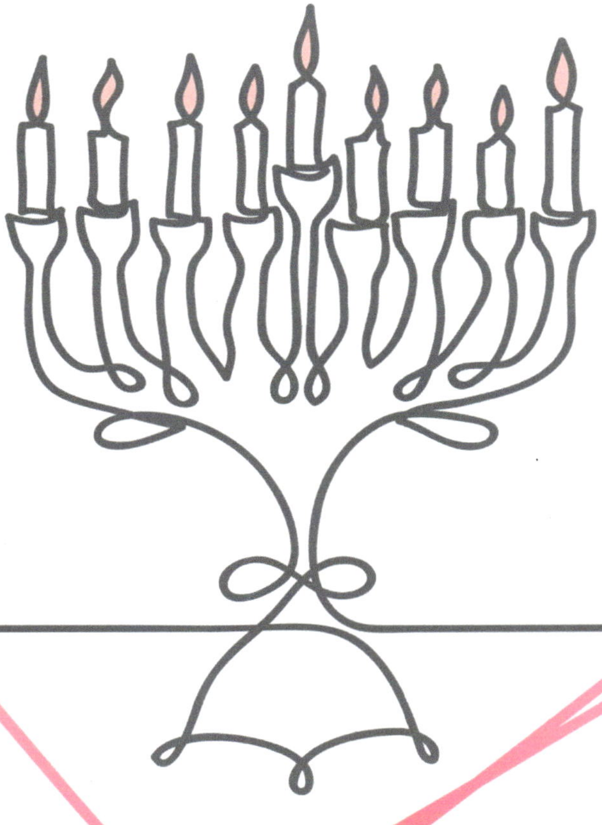

Cheese Latkes with Variations

Brenda

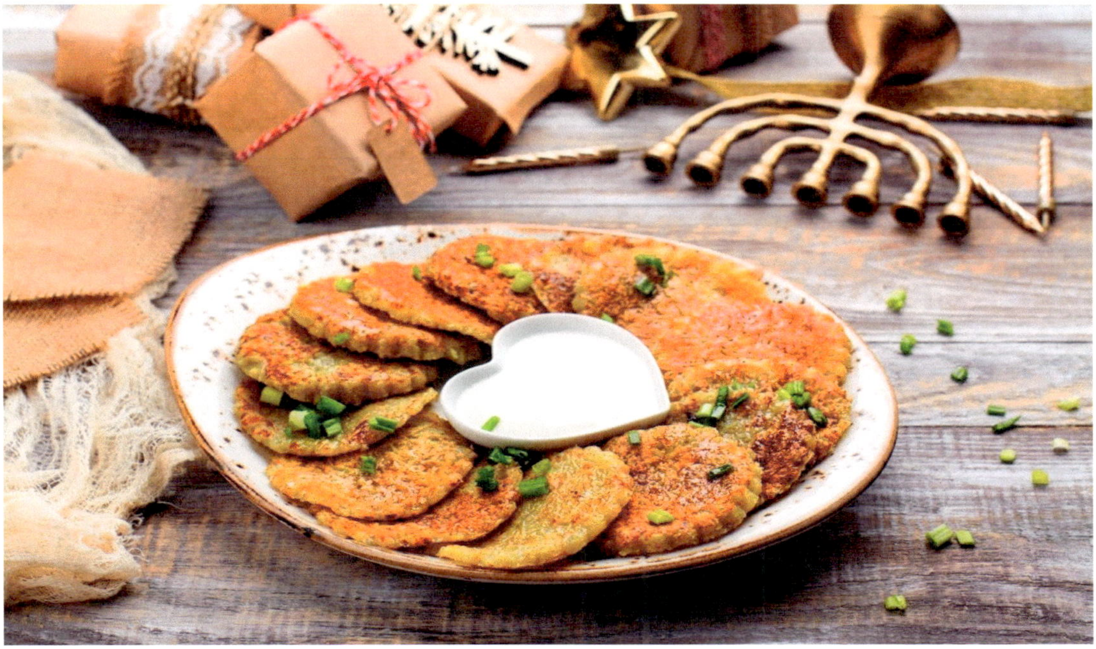

Bring Back the Cheese Latke!

Before the introduction of the potato, famine and poverty, Chanukah was primarily a dairy festival. Salted cheese was the preferred basis for latkes because cheese and wine was associated with the Jewish heroine Judith who was beautiful, brave and resourceful! She did what the men in her town were afraid to do - confront and conquer an overwhelming invading army! How did she do it? With cheese and oil and lots of wine. Her beauty and culinary skills overcame an army of men whose only vulnerability was their appetites.

Anyhow, cheese latkes are the original latkes. And delicious they are. I introduced them a few years ago to my grandchildren who love them and ask for them even when it is not Chanukah. I make them wait at least until winter to keep it special.

Here is the base recipe for cheese latkes:

Cheese Latke Base Recipe

Servings: 10 latkes (using # 30 1 ⅞ inch food scoop. 1 oz.)

Ingredients:

3 eggs
2 teaspoon psyllium husks
½ teaspoon of baking powder (cornstarch free, aluminium free, gluten free)
8.8 oz. l 250 g of pressed ricotta or cottage cheese full fat (check for gluten and emulsifiers)

Method:

1. Blend the eggs, psyllium husks and baking powder in a food processor
2. Add pressed ricotta cheese and blend some more
3. Let chill in fridge for one hour.

This is your base batter. You can divide this into smaller portions to make different variations. The only rule is that you can't use meat or poultry based fat - only vegetable or nut based oil for frying. Ghee or butter is okay.

Gluten free option | Nut free | Nightshade free | Lacto/Ovo Vegetarian

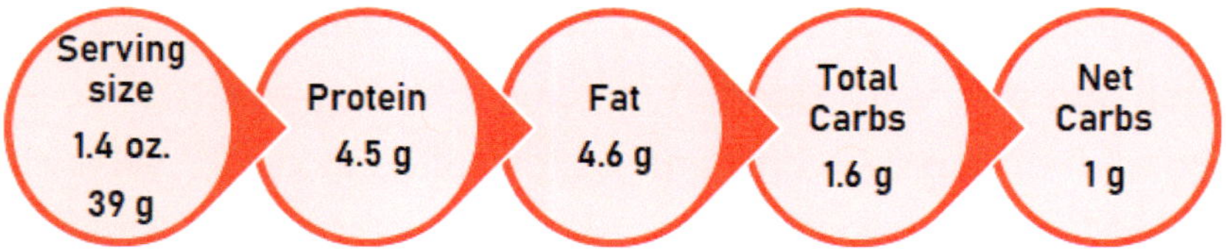

Dessert Latkes with Dairy

Servings: 6

Ingredients:

Using 1/2 of the basic recipe
15 drops of liquid stevia, or skip the sweetener altogether
1 tablespoon sour cream* or whipped heavy cream*
1 tablespoon berries such as raspberries or strawberries or blueberries**
or
1 tablespoon sugar-free applesauce
Oil of avocado, almond, light extra virgin olive, refined coconut (not vegetable oil)

Method:

1. Heat the frying pan to medium heat with the oil to ¼ inch on the bottom of the pan. (Drop a ½ teaspoon into oil to test, it should sizzle but not smoke.)
2. Drop 2 tablespoon | 40 g latke batter into the oil - gently sizzle.
3. Allow the bottom to brown slowly. When small holes appear in the top turn over and brown the other side.
4. Drain latkes – approximately 2 g of oil absorb into each latke.
5. Serve with a few berries, and a dollop of full fat sour cream or full fat whipped heavy cream. Or with a tablespoon of sugar-free applesauce.

Your non- keto friends and relatives can add maple syrup, honey or whatever! Enjoy your way - ketolicious! Don't forget to light the candles and enjoy the Oil and Light!

Substitutions:

People with dairy intolerance to A1 casein in cow's milk can try 250g goat cheese (chevron) which has the A2 protein (check label) and is generally better tolerated.

*Check for emulsifiers, and allergen list for gluten.

**Blueberries have been used in the macro count, raspberries would be lower in carbs. If using unsweetened applesauce add on 0.5 g carbs per serving.

Gluten free option | Nut free | Nightshade free | Lacto/Ovo/Vegetarian

Serving size	Protein	Fat	Total Carbs	Net Carbs
1.4 oz 39 g	3.8 g	6.3 g	1.7 g	1.1 g

Savoury Latkes

Servings: 6 Latkes

Ingredients:

1/2 of the basic cheese latke recipe
1 tablespoon finely minced dill
1 tablespoon finely minced green onion
Oil of avocado, almond, light extra virgin olive, refined coconut (not vegetable oil)
1 tablespoon of sour cream (optional, included in macro count)

Variations: Substitute your favorite herb for dill or onion: For example : parsley, coriander, fresh tarragon.

Method:

1. Heat the frying pan to medium heat with the oil to ¼ inch on the bottom of the pan. (Drop a ½ teaspoon into oil to test, it should sizzle but not smoke.)
2. Drop 2 tablespoon | 40 g latke batter into the oil - gently sizzle.
3. Allow the bottom to brown slowly. When small holes appear in the top turn over and brown the other side.
4. Drain latkes – approximately 2 g of oil absorb into each latke.
5. Serve with a dollop of sour cream, as a side to pan fried fish or on its own.

Gluten free option | Nut free | Nightshade free | Lacto/Ovo/Vegetarian

Serving size	Protein	Fat	Total Carbs	Net Carbs
1.3 oz 38 g	3.8 g	6.3 g	1.5 g	0.9 g

Beet Latkes with Smoked Salmon and Herbed Cream Cheese

Servings: 1

Ingredients:

1 x beet latke, cooked (see recipe below)
1 slice | 1 oz |28 g of smoked salmon
¼ cup softened cream cheese*
¼ cup sour cream*
1 teaspoon dill, finely chopped
1 teaspoon parsley, finely chopped
1 teaspoon green onion, finely chopped

Method:

1. Place a cooked beet latke on your serving plate.
2. Mix the cream cheese with the herbs.
3. Add a dollop (approx. 1 tablespoon) of the herbed cream cheese.
4. Top with the smoked salmon.

*Check for emulsifiers and allergen list for gluten.

Gluten free option | Nut free | Nightshade free

Serving size	Protein	Fat	Total Carbs	Net Carbs
1.2 oz 35 g	2 g	5.5 g	2 g	1.6 g

Pan Fried Salmon Patties, also known as Rissoles in England

Servings: 6 for starters, 3 for main course

These were one of my husband's specialities. Originally they were made with matzoh meal as were the veggie latkes. But with my need to stay gluten free we experimented with other options. The function of the matzoh meal, a very dry wheat based meal, was to bind up the egg and other ingredients so that the mixture stays together during the frying process. The matzoh meal soaks up and binds the liquid or moisture in the mix. After much experiment, some of it quite awful (i.e chia seed, flax meal, etc.). We/ I hit on the combination of psyllium husk powder and tiger nut flour. Almond flour could also be used. These ingredients bind without sliminess, and the flavor doesn't overpower.

Ingredients:

1 can of Wild Red Sockeye Salmon. 213 g 7.5 oz, drained.
½ teaspoon psyllium husk powder
1 tablespoon tiger nut flour (or finely ground almond flour)
1 egg
1 teaspoon finely chopped green onion
1 teaspoon finely chopped dill
1 teaspoon finely chopped parsley
Oil of avocado, almond, light extra virgin olive, refined coconut (not vegetable oil)

Method:

1. Place all ingredients in a small bowl. Mix thoroughly.
2. Chill in the fridge for at least 1 hour.
3. Heat the frying pan to medium heat with the oil to ¼ inch on the bottom of the pan. (Drop a ½ teaspoon into oil to test, it should sizzle but not smoke.)

4. Drop 2 tablespoon l 40 g salmon mixture into the oil - gently sizzle.
5. Allow the bottom to brown slowly then top turn over and brown the other side.
6. Drain and serve.
7. Drain latkes – approximately 2 g of oil absorb into each latke.
8. You can serve with any side (not included in macro count).

Gluten free option | Nightshade free

Note: Macro count based on 6 servings as a starter

Serving size	Protein	Fat	Total Carbs	Net Carbs
1.7 oz 49 g	9.1 g	6.1 g	2.4 g	0.9 g

Vegetarian Latkes

serve with vegetarian, meat or dairy/fish

Beet Latkes

Servings: 6 latkes

Ingredients:

1 egg
1 teaspoon psyllium husk powder
I medium beet (beetroot) peeled and grated to fill 1 cup loosely packed
1 cup grated zucchini to fill 1 cup measure loosely packed (see prep instruction for zucchini latkes)
2 tablespoon finely minced onion - red, or sweet
Oil of avocado, almond, light extra virgin olive, refined coconut (not vegetable oil)
I teaspoon toasted caraway seeds (optional)

Method:

1. Follow the instruction for broccoli slaw latkes (recipe below) with the following substitutions.
2. Use grated beet (beetroot) and zucchini instead of broccoli slaw.
3. Parcook for 2.5 minutes with the onion and caraway (optional).

These latkes can be used for Beet Latkes with Salmon and herbed Cream cheese.

Gluten free option | Nut free | Nightshade free | Lacto/Ovo/Vegetarian

Serving size	Protein	Fat	Total Carbs	Net Carbs
2.2 oz 62 g	1.8 g	2.9 g	5.8 g	3.6 g

Broccoli Slaw Latkes

Servings: 6 latkes

Ingredients:

1 egg
1 teaspoon psyllium husk powder
2 loosely packed cups I 170 g of prepared broccoli slaw (I use President's Choice in Canada)
2 tablespoon minced onion
Salt or seasoned salt to taste (I use Herbamare)
Oil of avocado, almond, light extra virgin olive, refined coconut (not vegetable oil)

Method:

1. Whisk egg and psyllium husk powder together. Set aside.
2. Parcook the broccoli slaw and onion together. I use a vegetable steamer in the microwave for 2 minutes - no water added.
3. Drain broccoli slaw and onion mixture - place veggies in a strainer and press out any excess water.
4. Fold into the egg and psyllium husk mixture. Let sit in fridge for about 1 hour. (or not if you are in a hurry).
5. Heat the frying pan to medium heat with the oil to ¼ inch on the bottom of the pan. (Drop a ½ teaspoon into oil to test, it should sizzle but not smoke.)
6. Drop 2 tablespoon I 40 g latke batter into the oil - gently sizzle.
7. Allow the bottom to brown slowly. When small holes appear in the top turn over and brown the other side.
8. Drain latkes – approximately 2 g of oil absorb into each latke.
9. You can put the cooked latkes in the oven on warm if you are waiting for other dishes to cook or get ready.

Serving Suggestions:

If you are serving with fish or dairy or vegetarian you can garnish with sour cream or with mayonnaise or aioli, or even a dill pickle tartar sauce (made with avocado oil mayonnaise). If you are serving with a meat dish stick to the mayonnaise based sauces or a guacamole dressing.

Gluten free option | Nut free | Nightshade free | Lacto/Ovo/Vegetarian

Serving size	Protein	Fat	Total Carbs	Net Carbs
1.4 oz 39 g	1.6 g	2.8 g	2.9 g	1.6 g

Zucchini Latkes

Servings: 6 latkes

Ingredients:

1 egg
1 teaspoon psyllium husk powder
2 or 3 small young zucchini, to make 2 cups loosely packed grated zucchini
2 tablespoon finely minced onion - red, or sweet
Oil for cooking - avocado, almond, light extra virgin olive, refined coconut (not vegetable oil)

Method:

1. Prepare the zucchini by slicing each one in half. Scoop out the inner core of pulp and baby seed. Grate using hand, crank or food processor grater; medium grate.
2. Follow the instruction for broccoli slaw latkes with the following substitutions. Use grated zucchini instead of broccoli slaw. Parcook for 1.5 minutes with the onion.

*You really do need to pay attention when you are cooking with oil. Consider it a form of meditation.

Gluten free option | Nut free | Nightshade free | Lacto/Ovo/Vegetarian

Serving size	Protein	Fat	Total Carbs	Net Carbs
1.9 oz 54 g	1.4 g	2.9 g	2.3 g	1.2 g

May this season
be festive & your
laughter be contagious

Ways to Navigate Social Pressures of Food & the Holidays

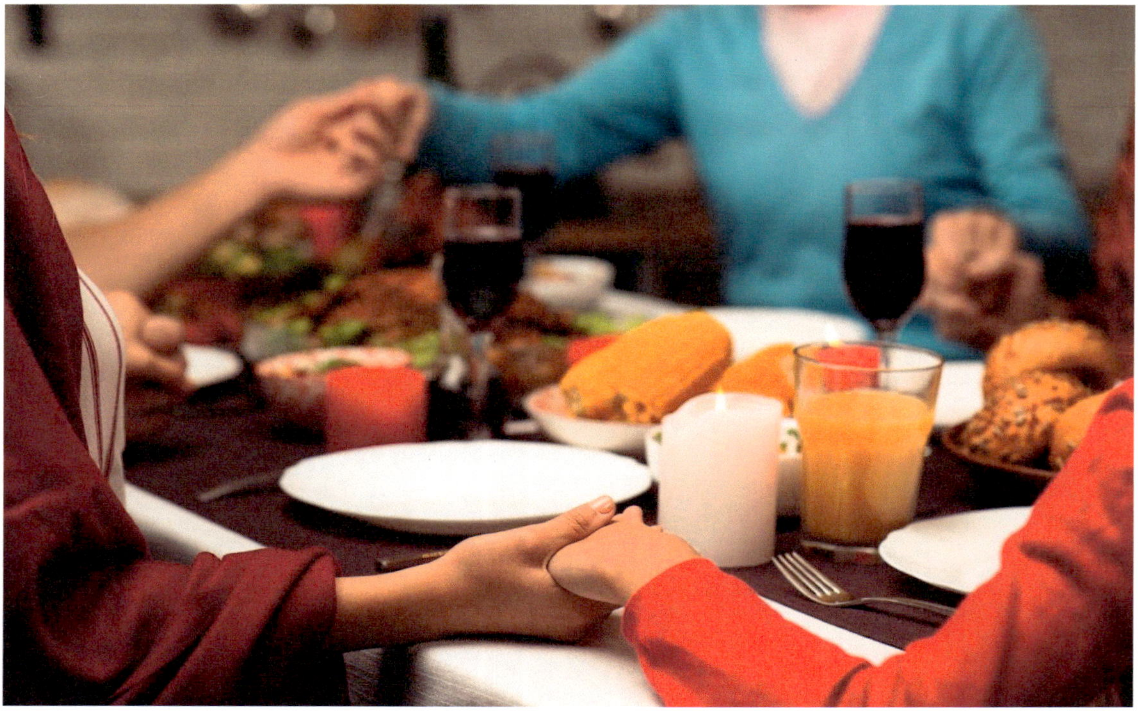

Holidays bring festivities and lots of gorgeous and tempting food surrounds us. Much like this family picture above, you will probably be in settings with "foods we don't eat!" Although holidays and celebrations tend to be centered around food, they can really be about connection with family and friends. With a bit of planning, you can come through the holidays remaining in ketosis. Whatever your food choices are, enjoy the fellowship, sharing and joy of the season. Here are some tips to help you stay on your eating plan through the holidays.

1. **Make an eating plan and stick to it:** Have some idea of what food choices will be at your destination. What foods do you plan to eat? Which ones will you avoid? What do you plan to do when faced with temptation? Alert others to give you support if you are worried you will need it.

2. **Let your host know your eating restrictions:** This will take the pressure off of you if you feel it would be impolite not to eat all the offerings. For instance, a host that has been warned that you won't eat anything with wheat can't be upset when you don't try some homemade pasta.
3. **Defensive Eating:** Eat something filling, maybe an entire meal, before going to a social event when you know food choices will be poor and/or very tempting. If you are full, resisting temptation will be easier. At the event, be sure to hold a beverage (preferably water, coffee or tea) to show that you are participating as much as you are able.
4. **Distraction:** Keep yourself busy! This won't be a problem if you are hosting a Holiday event, but you may need something to distract you from enticing smells from the kitchen when you are away from home. Offer to help with decorations or last-minute trips to the store. You may like working on a craft or other Holiday project, entertaining the children with games and stories, or otherwise being helpful to your hosts.
5. **Offer to bring a dish** so you know there will be something you can eat. This can be a great opportunity to showcase the delicious foods you get to eat everyday as part of ketogenic eating. You may find that your contributions are gone very quickly!
6. If **Holiday desserts** will be the greatest temptation to you and the most likely to derail you from your eating plan, use this opportunity to impress everyone with a spectacular traditional dessert that is low carb. Bringing a dessert that you can enjoy will help you from feeling deprived.
7. **Have a ready explanation** for your food choices and/or refusals that you feel comfortable with. Remember, you don't have to offer any explanation if you aren't asked. Here are some examples:
   - "My doctor has put me on a special diet."
   - "I'm testing to see if I'm allergic to (chocolate, dairy, sugar, wheat, etc) so I can't have that."
   - "I've started a special way of eating and have already lost XX pounds, so I don't want to quit now. I know you'll support me on this!"

8. **Redirection:** When offered a dish that is off your eating plan, simply reply "No, thank you" and immediately offer a different topic of discussion. This is a good option if you don't want to engage in a nutrition debate.

   For example:

   "No, thank you. I hear you just returned from vacation. Tell me about your trip!"

9. **Fill your plate up with foods you *can* eat.** A full plate isn't as obvious as one that has very little on it. You may find that no one notices at all that you aren't having any rolls or mashed potatoes.

Remember, you can eat well, stay in ketosis, enjoy your food, your family, your friends, your holidays AND take care of yourself. You are worth it!

Happy Holidays!

Leslyn

Leslyn Keith, OTD, CLT-LANA
Director of Research
The Lipedema Project
leslyn@lipedema-simplified.org

"The main thing to making food precious is to quiet and calm ourselves enough to let the experience touch our hearts. So in a way what becomes precious is our capacity to slow down and actually receive things. It's the gift of our own consciousness." ~Edward Espe Brown

Peace

Joy

& LOVE

from all of us
to all of you!

Made in the USA
Las Vegas, NV
10 November 2026

57843116R00093